Nurse Dorothea presents Social Media and Social Networking with Their Benefits and Disadvantages

Authored by Michael Dow, RN, MS, MHA, MSM

Illustrations by Lindsay Roberts, M.Ed, BFA

Nurse Dorothea presents Social Media and Social Networking with Their Benefits and Disadvantages

Copyright © 2024 by Dow Creative Enterprises, LLC

All rights reserved

First Edition

ISBN 979-8-9905577-6-5

Printed by Lulu

Published by Dow Creative Enterprises®

Dow Creative Enterprises, LLC

PO Box 15357

Tucson, AZ 85708

Library of Congress Control Number: 2024922397

Dow Creative Enterprises® is a federally registered trademark with the United States Patent and Trademark Office.

Help Civilization Reach Its Potential® is a federally registered trademark with the United States Patent and Trademark Office.

Table of Contents

Title	Page Number
Dedication	vi
Part 1	1
Part 2	123
References	242
About the Illustrator	247
About the Author	249
Other Books by DCE	251

Dedication

The Nurse Dorothea book series is dedicated to Dorothea Dix. Her work in the 1800s helped people with mental illness live a more dignified life. She spent decades lobbying government officials to create state hospitals for the mentally ill. One person can make a difference.

Michael

Part 1

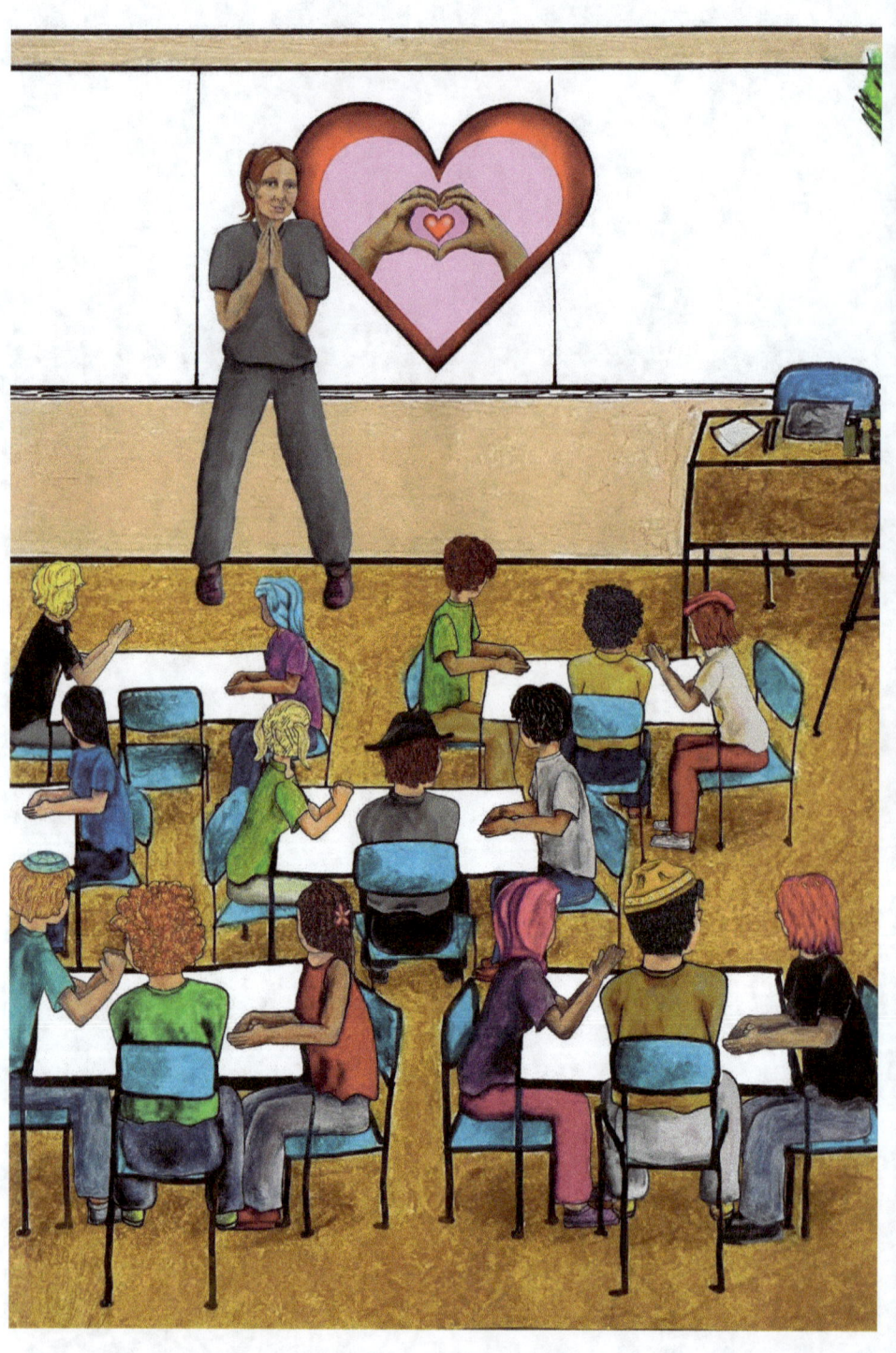

"Hi everyone. My name is Nurse Dorothea. Thank you for coming to the after-school club on mental health. I hope to provide you with some tools to manage your emotions and navigate life's challenges. Mental health is complicated because there are so many things that can affect it. This class was created to show that it is ok to talk about your mental health with others as well as to give you ideas to improve your mental health."

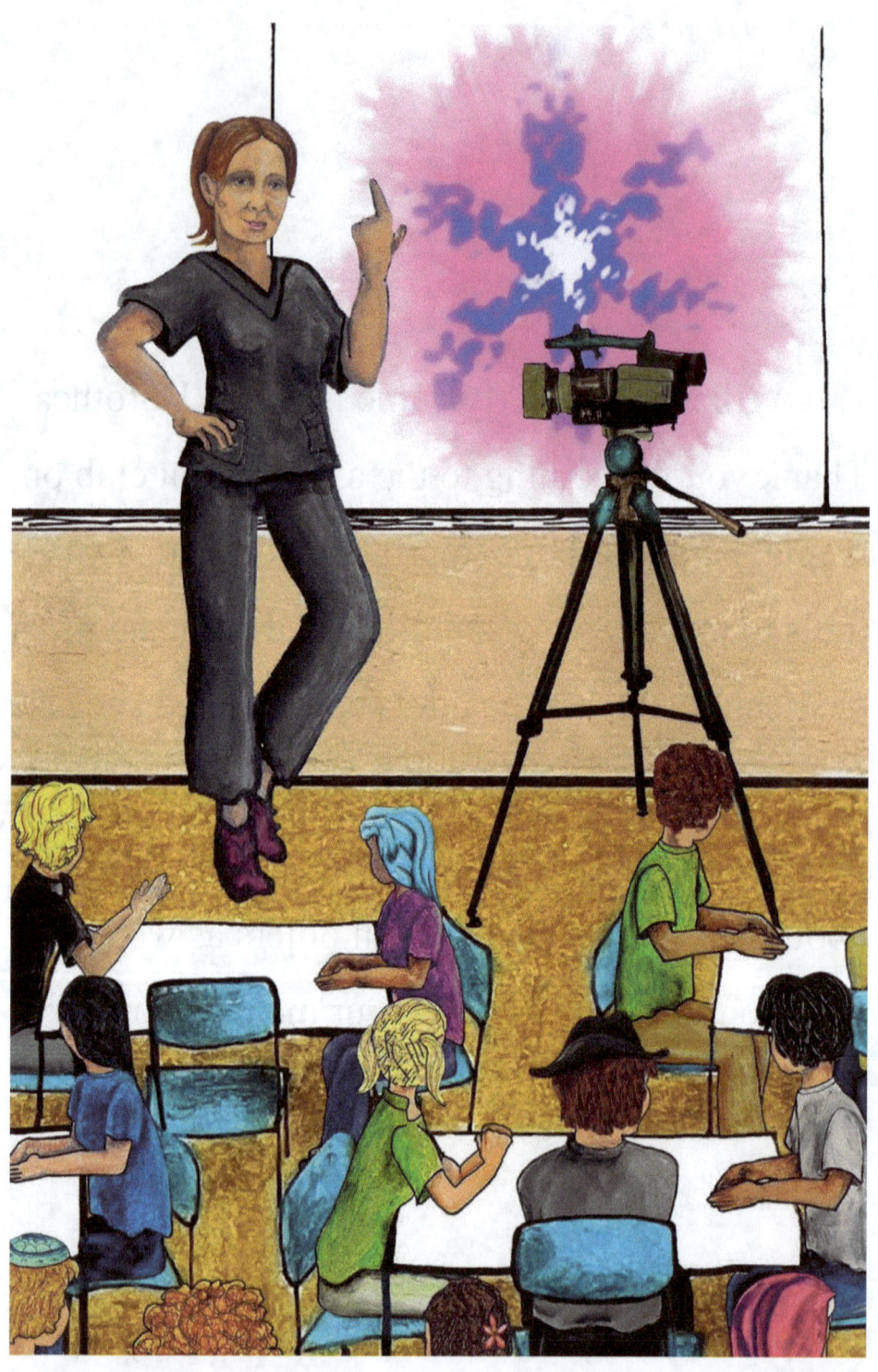

"We will be recording this session. People in the future will get to experience the same things you will today. Sometimes, I will speak to people watching this show or reading the future book about the class. This is an interactive class, and I want you all to ask questions as you have them. We will stop sometimes and discuss things with each other. If you are watching the show or reading the book, then I want YOU all to also discuss the questions and topics with those in the room. This book is an experience, and you will only get the full experience by talking with others. Please take breaks from the show as you need to since this will be a long discussion."

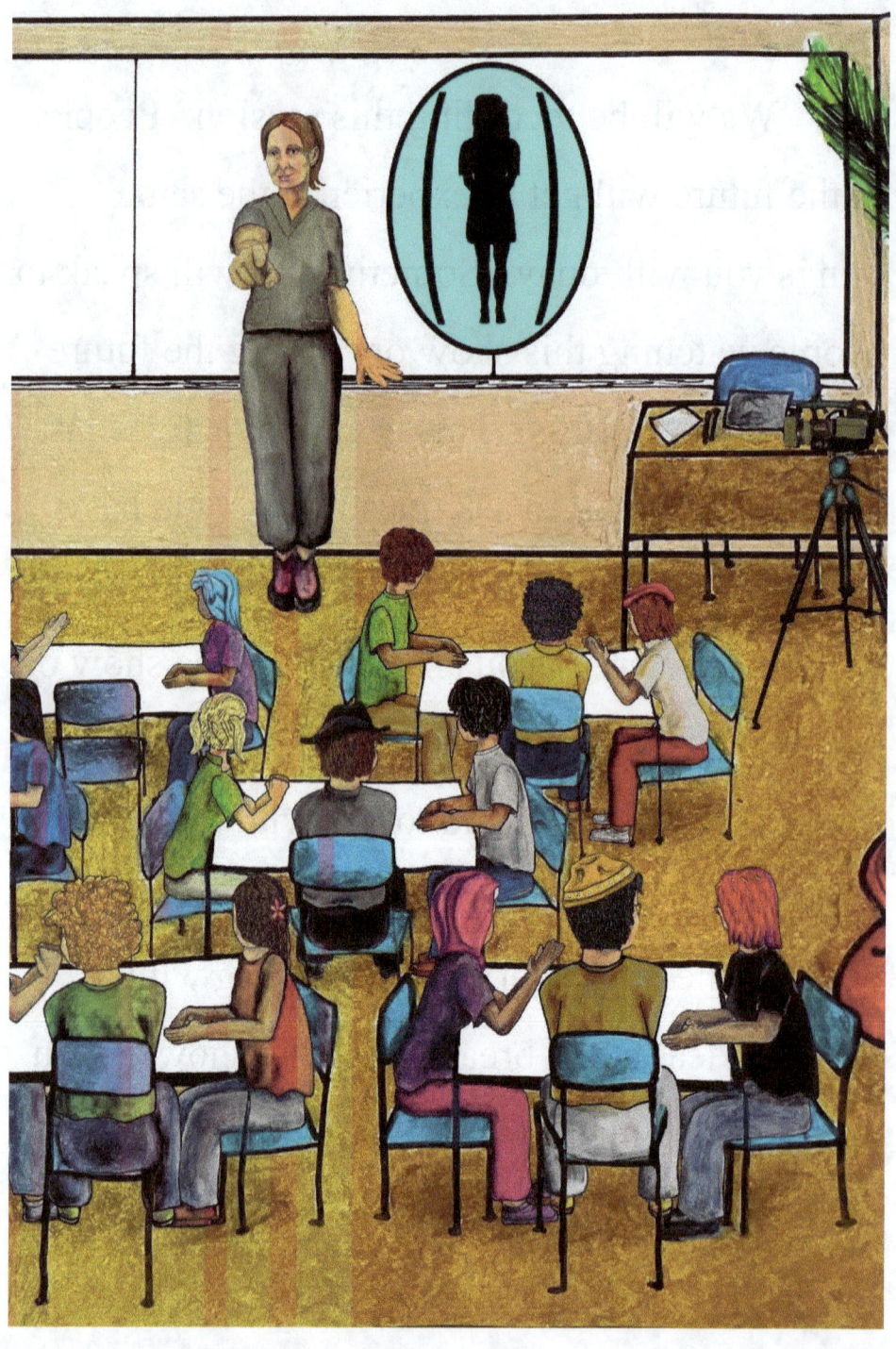

"If you are watching the show or reading this book alone, that is ok. Please take the time right now to get out a journal. I want those doing this class by themselves to write down responses to questions I will ask so that you participate like all the others. Sometimes, we need to address some mental health issues alone, so that is why it is ok to do this class by yourself. We are on a journey that is ultimately our own, but it is always nice to have people alongside us to help us in the bad times and share our joy in the good times."

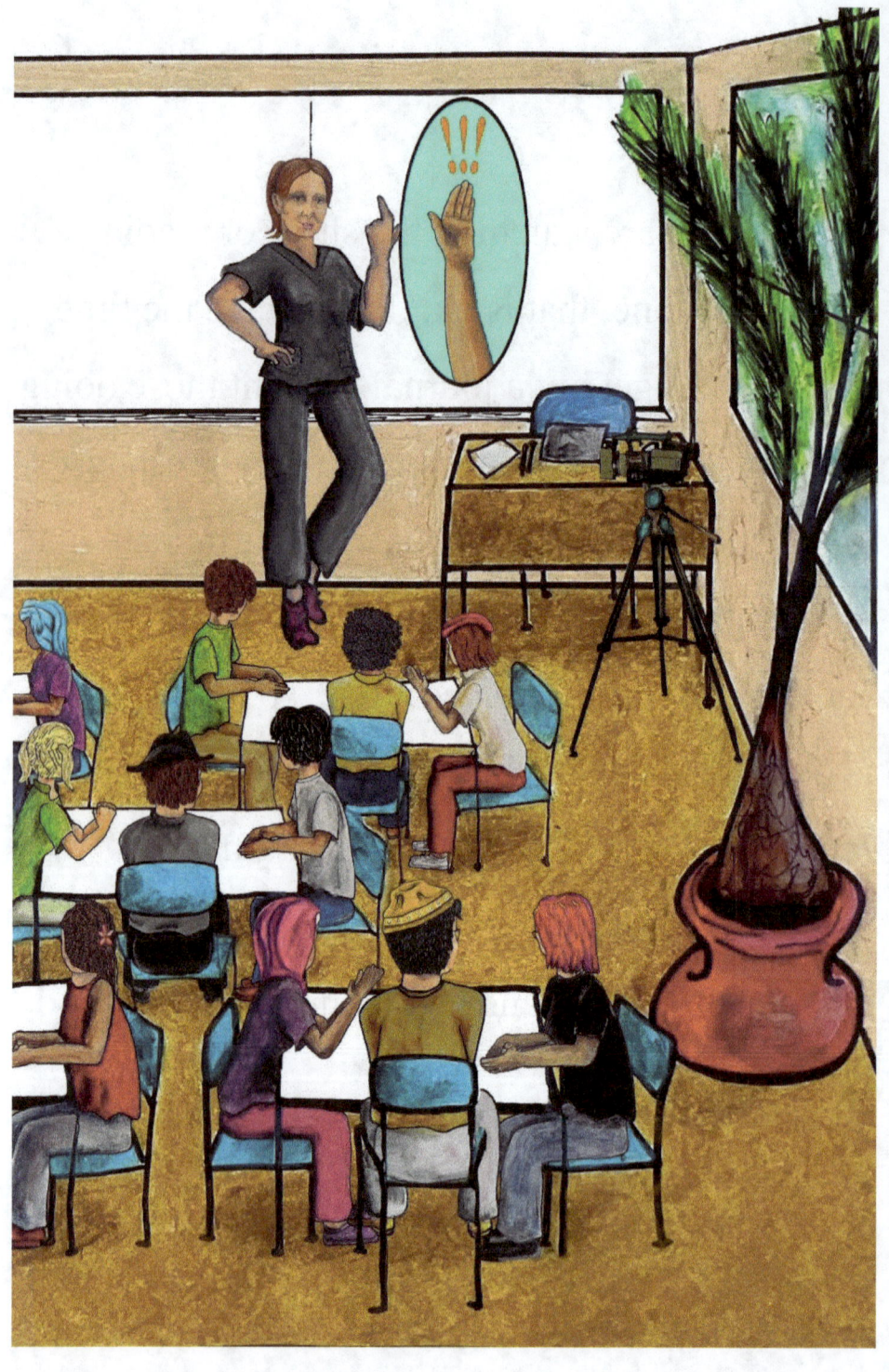

"The main rule for the class is to respect others. If someone has a question, we are to be quiet and let them speak. Raise your hand if you have a question, and I will call on you. Respecting everyone is important since we can learn from everyone."

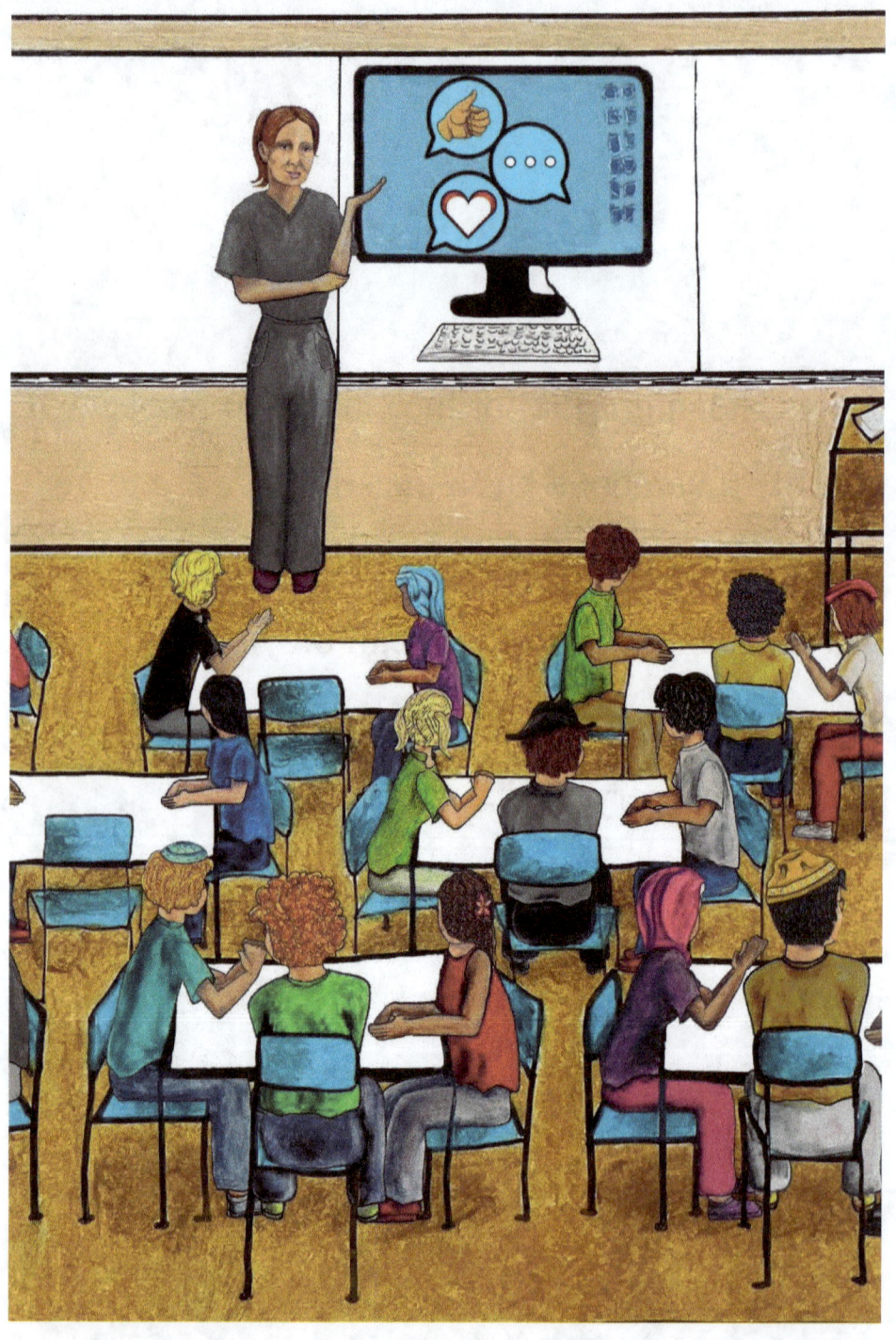

"Today's class will be about social media and social networking. Social media is defined by Oxford Languages as 'websites and applications that enable users to create and share content or to participate in social networking.' Social media is a permanent part of the digital world that we live in. We need social networking to get questions answered easily and to help in our careers. Those of us who have already been using social media have probably been cyberbullied or had negative reactions to something that we have posted which may have frustrated or upset us. Since social media is part of our world, we need to understand how best to use it. We should be aware of its benefits and disadvantages. Our world is complex, and we need to learn to effectively manage the tools that we use to live instead of letting a tool manage our life."

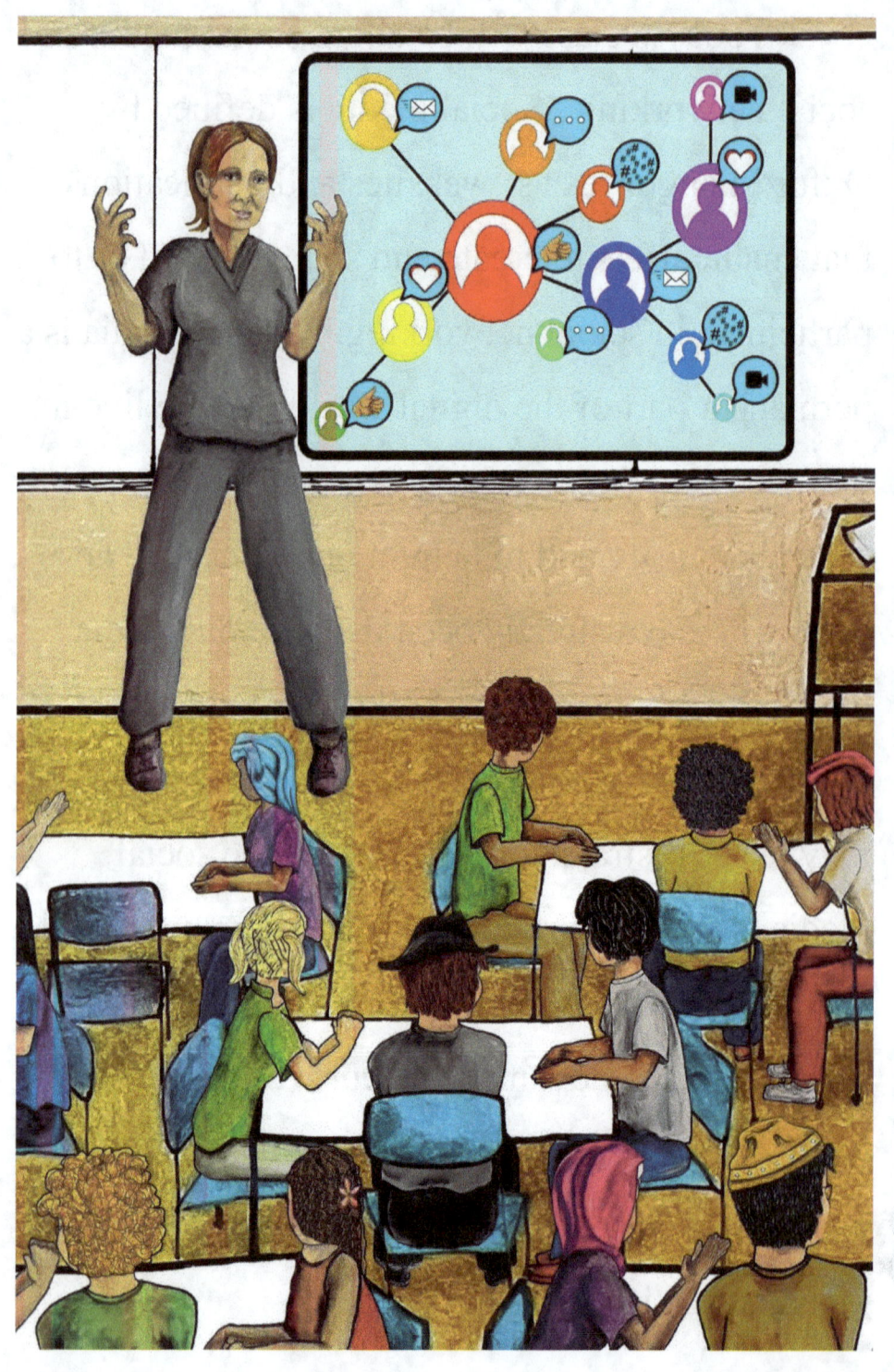

"The Encyclopedia Britannica states that social media is 'a form of mass media communications on the internet, like websites for social networking and microblogging, through which users share information, ideas, personal messages, and other content.' Social networking is when users build communities among themselves, while social media focuses on building an audience."

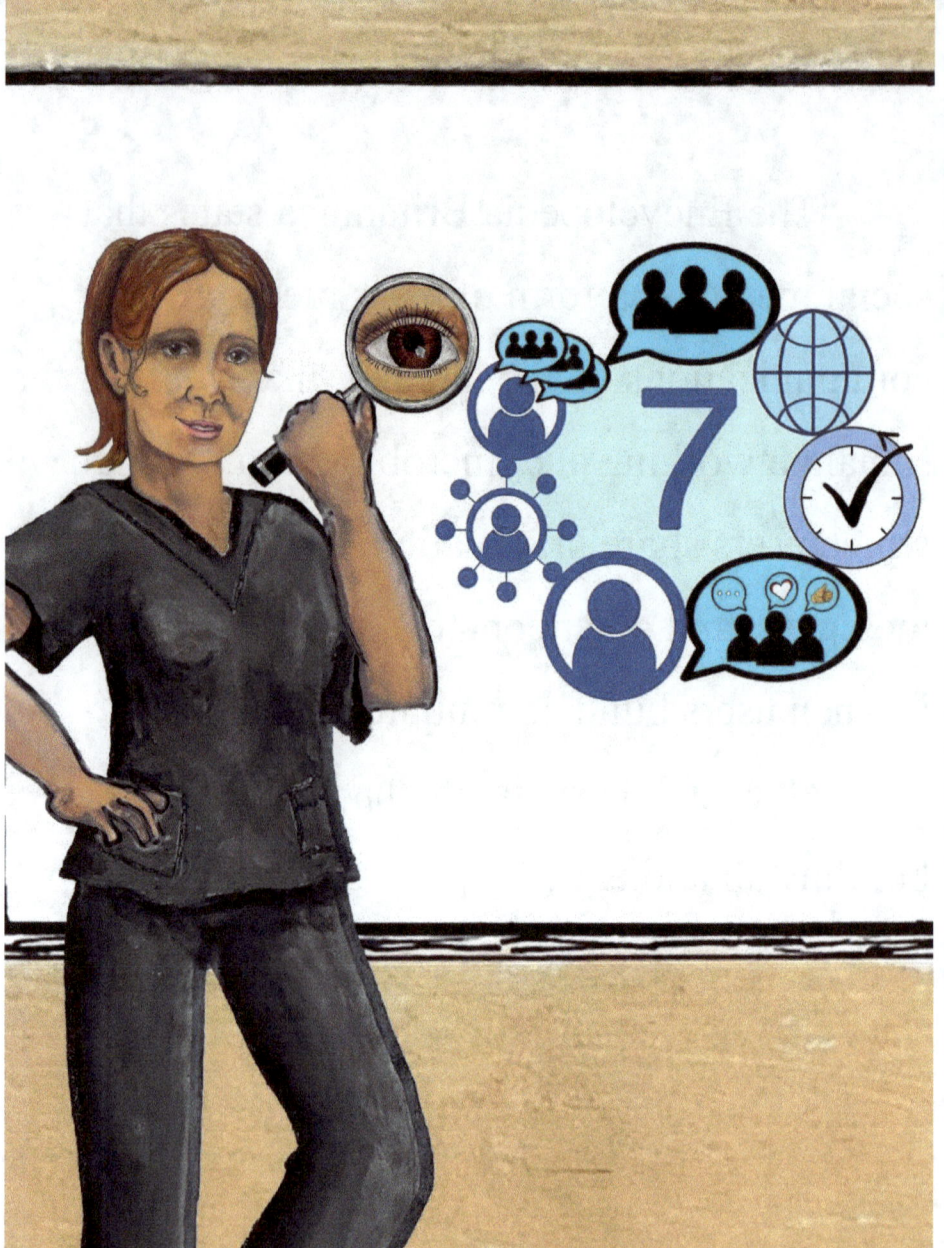

"Some websites may not seem like social media because they act like search engines or other things. They may still encourage communication and help people create profiles to share personal information. There are seven characteristics that define something as social media."

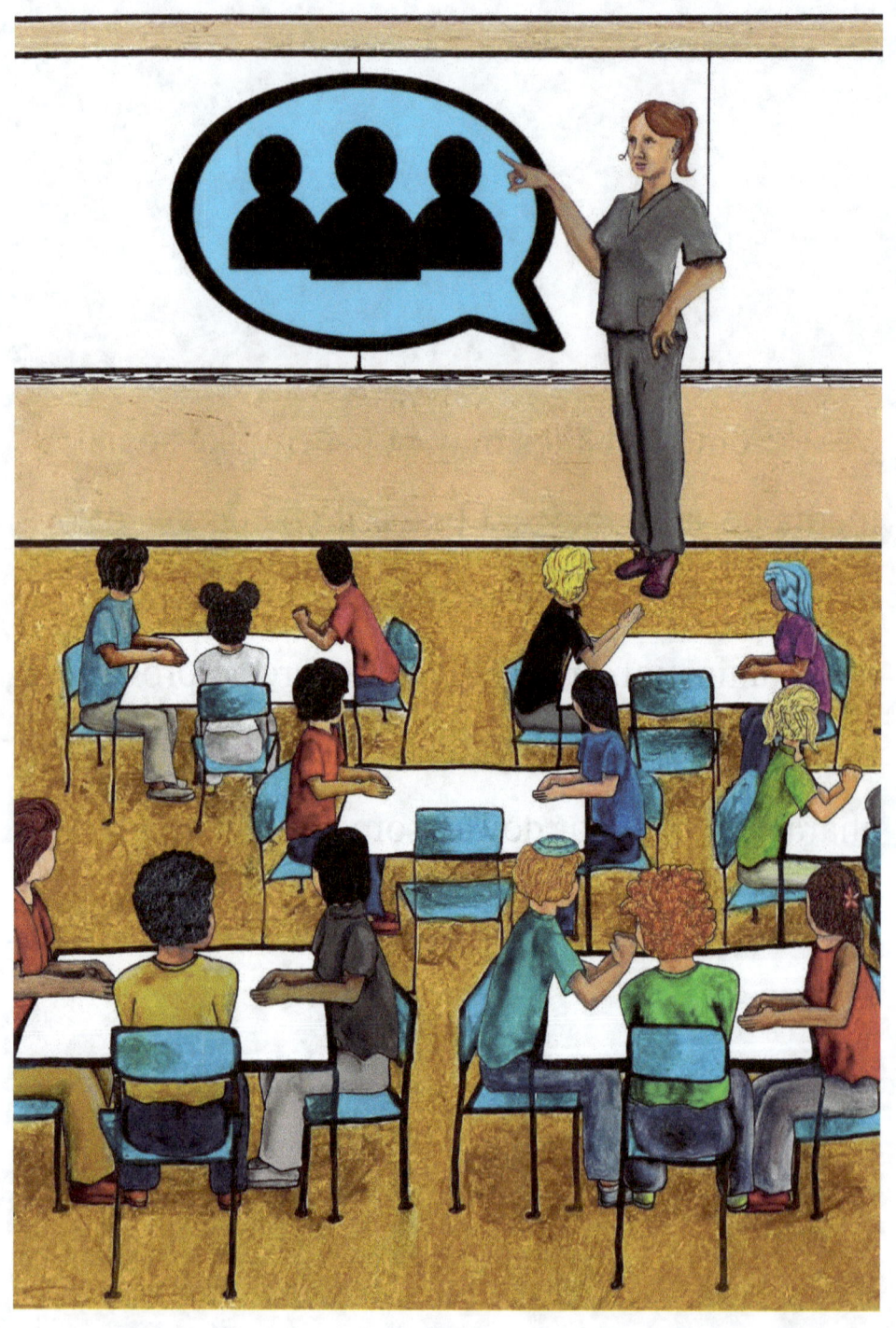

"The first characteristic is called participatory. This means that users can interact with others. It might be as simple as leaving a comment under a video so that others can read your opinion."

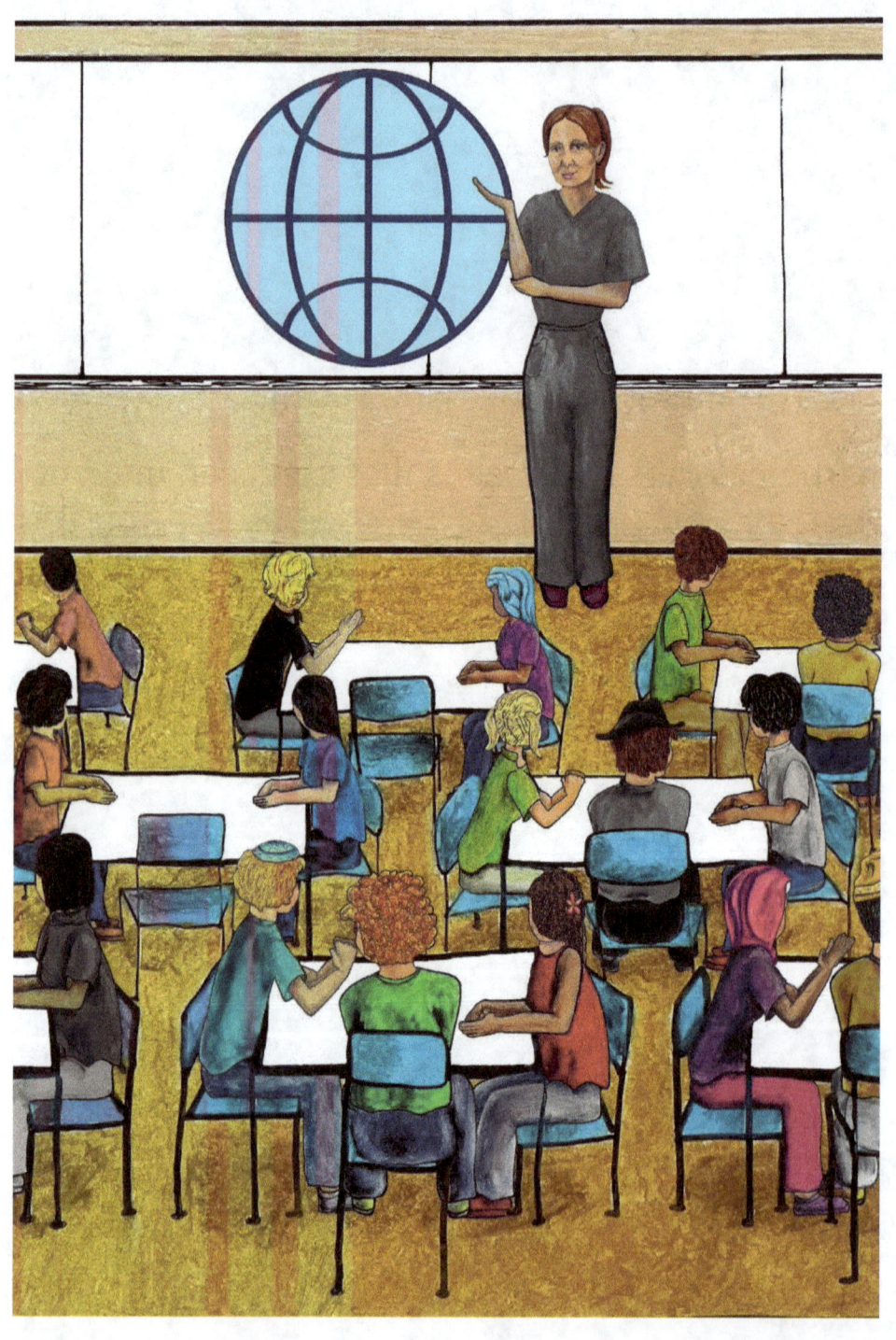

"The second characteristic is called being public. Social media is public, meaning anyone can see the content that you leave. This is why people should be cautious about what content they want to post or display. For example, you may not want to input your date of birth, full name, and address, because that means others will know that information and could use that to steal your identity and cause you financial problems by charging things in your name."

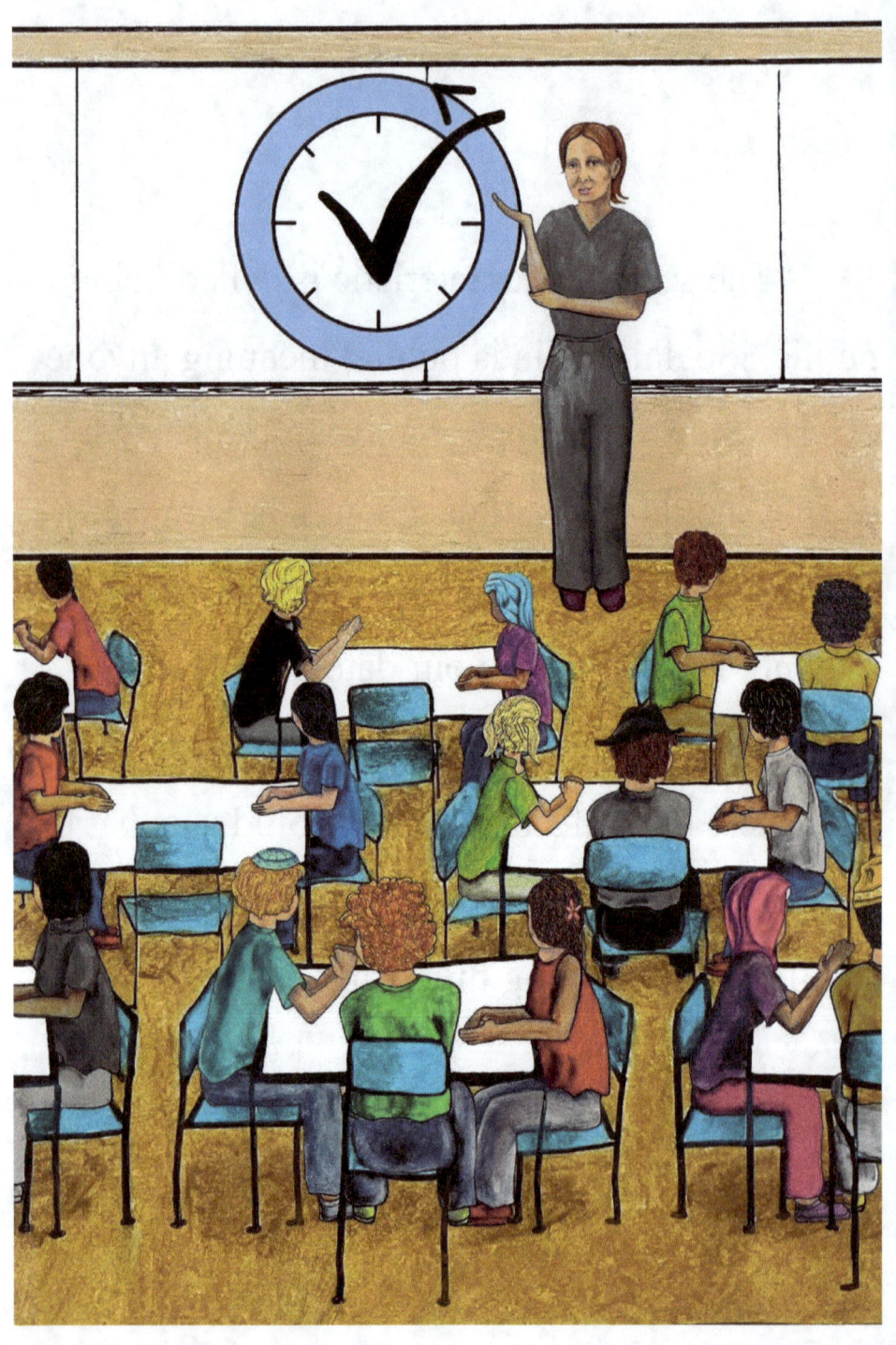

"The third thing about social media is that it's in real-time. Users of social media can post things immediately for others to see and read other people's content immediately after they post it."

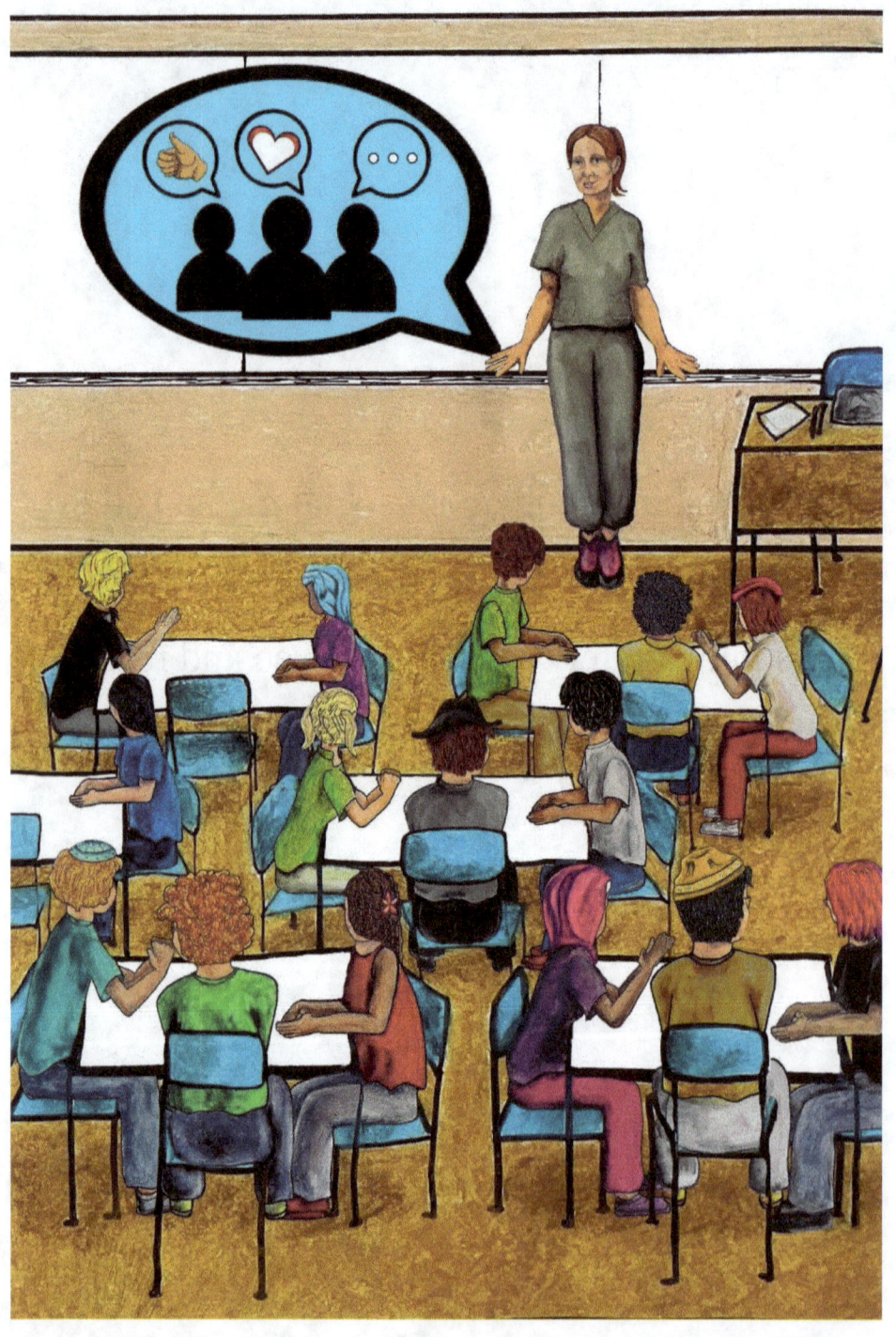

"The fourth characteristic is that it's user-generated content. Users are producers of the content, which means they are partly in control of creating a sub-culture because they determine what is posted and learned from each other."

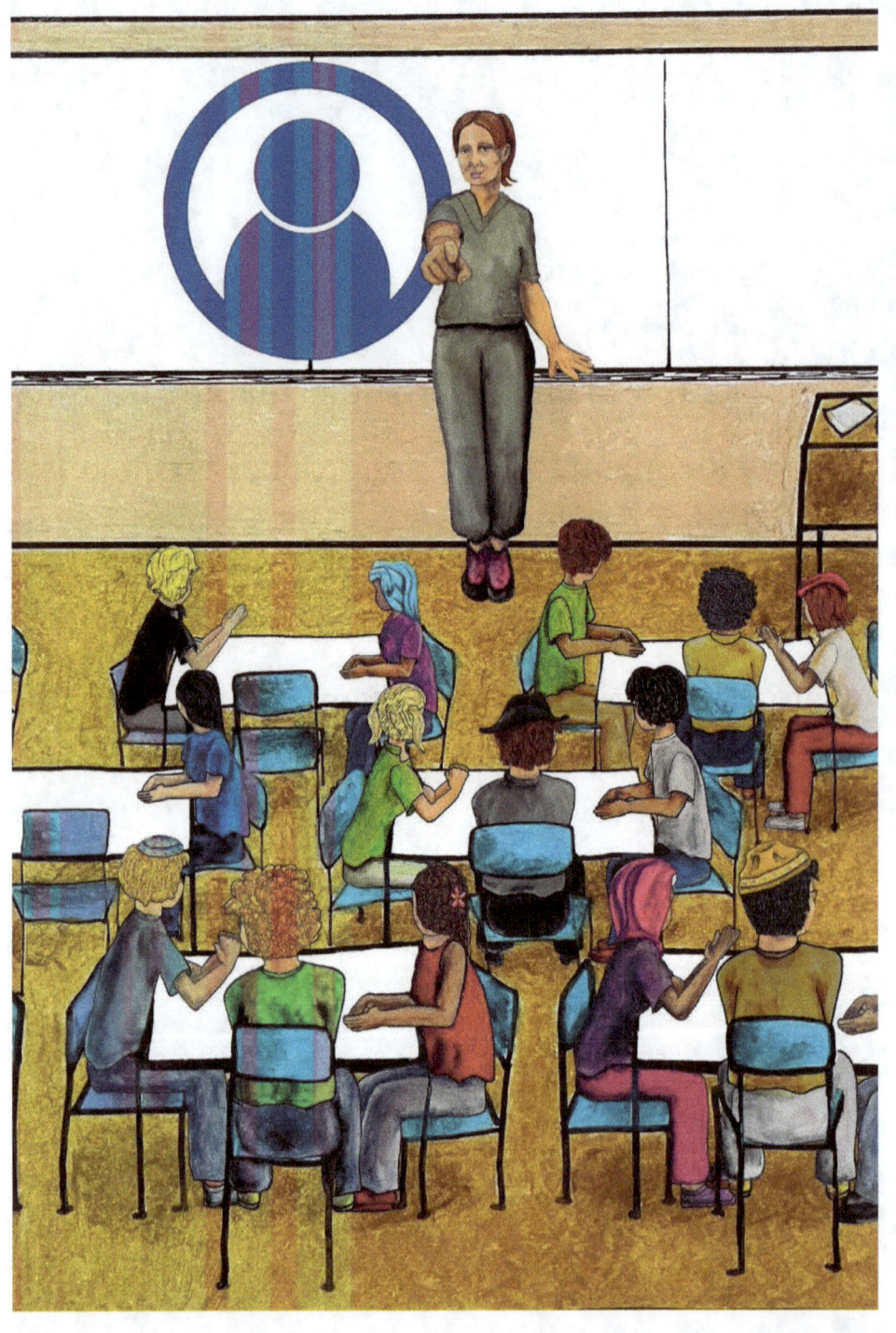

"The fifth part of what social media is involves user profiles. A user profile allows people to share information about themselves. They might even create an avatar or an image of something that is supposed to represent themselves on the website or application."

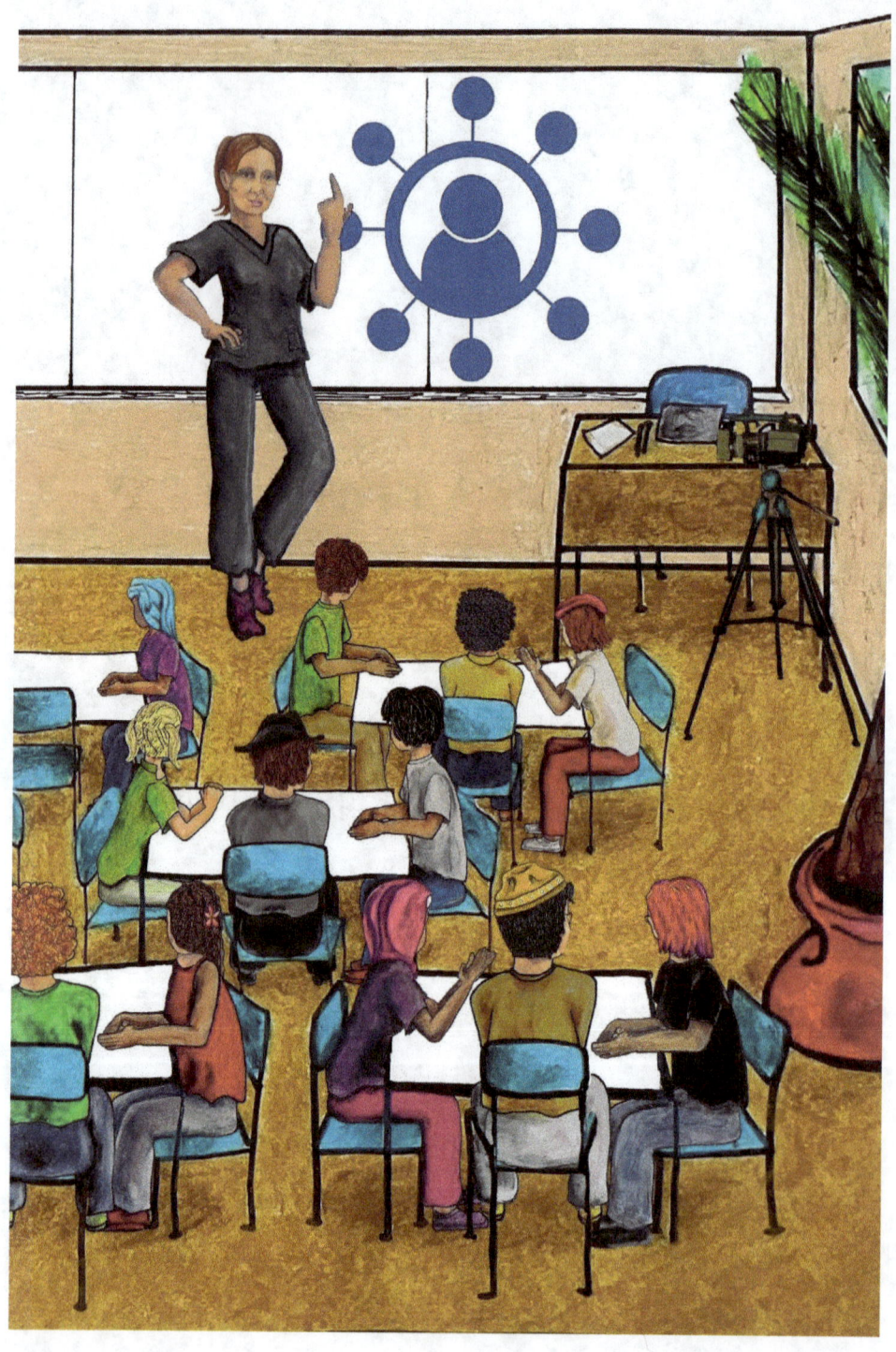

"The sixth characteristic is social networks. Social media helps to create social networking where groups of people share interests and communicate with others digitally. A social network can revolve around any type of interest like a favorite movie, favorite hobby, or favorite part of a culture such as food."

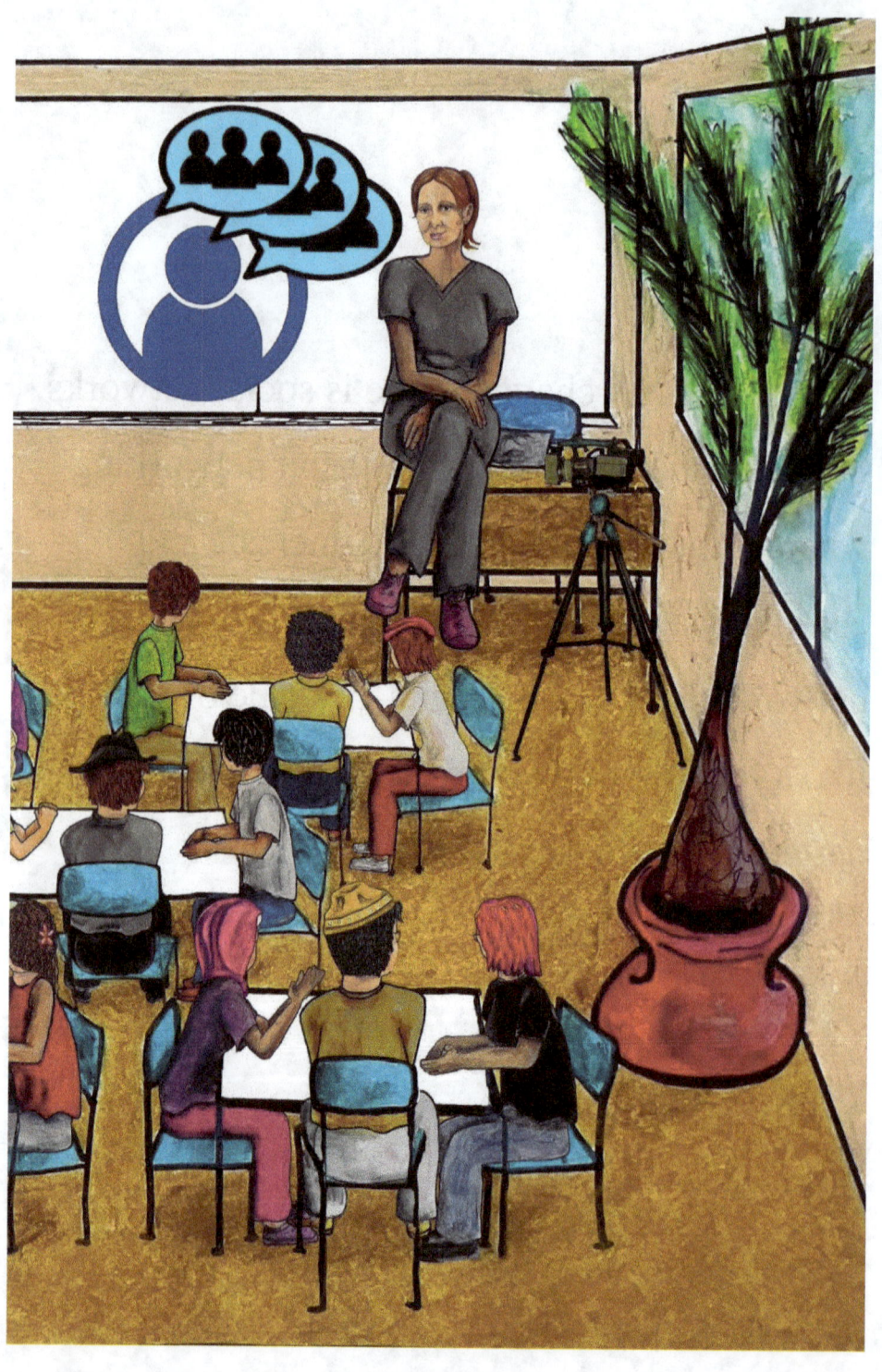

"The last characteristic of social media is that it's a one-to-many communication. A user can communicate an idea to many different people all at once."

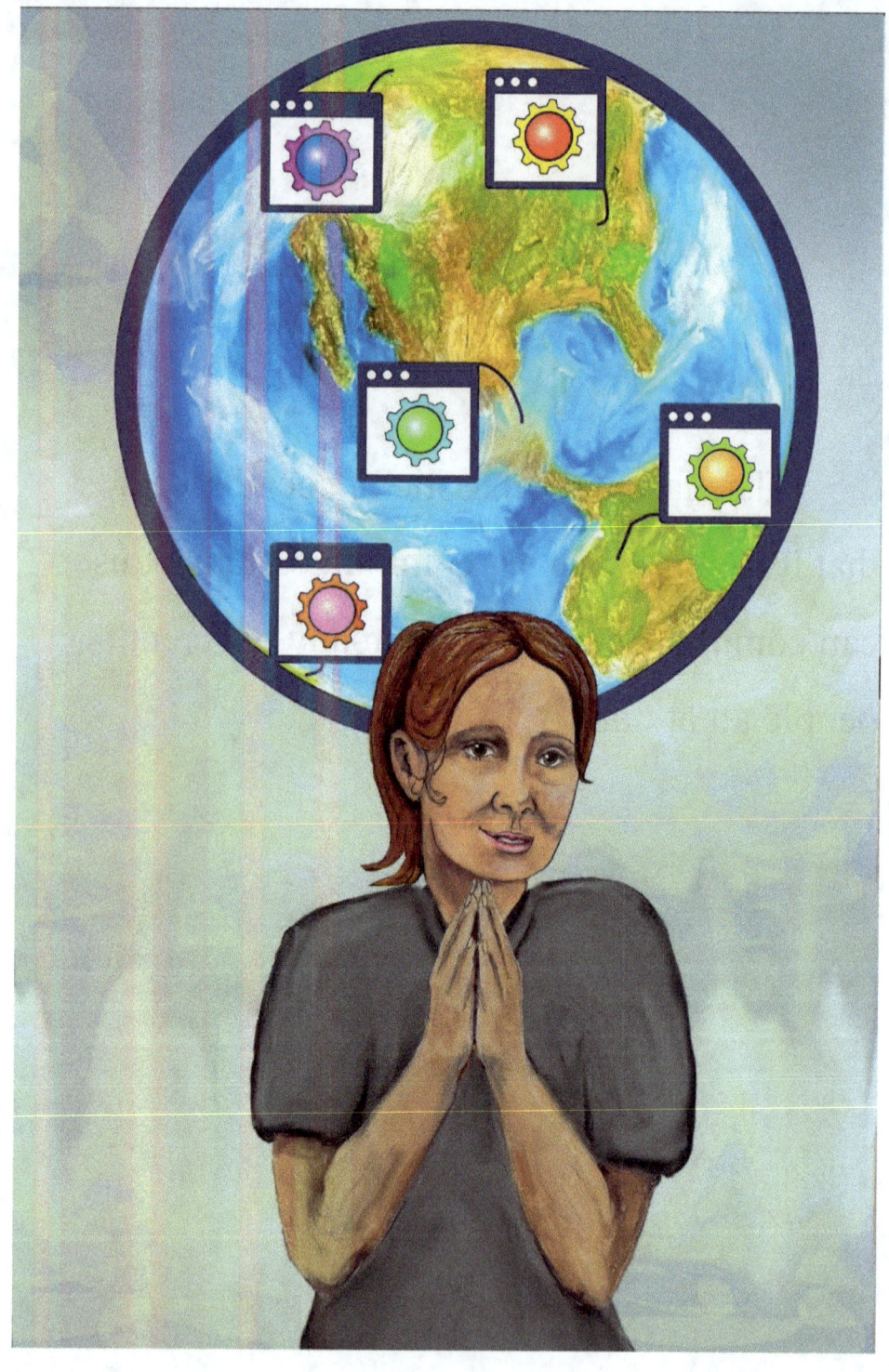

"In order to not advertise specific social media platforms, we won't discuss certain popular apps. Some are popular in certain countries, and others are popular in various categories of the population such as specific age groups."

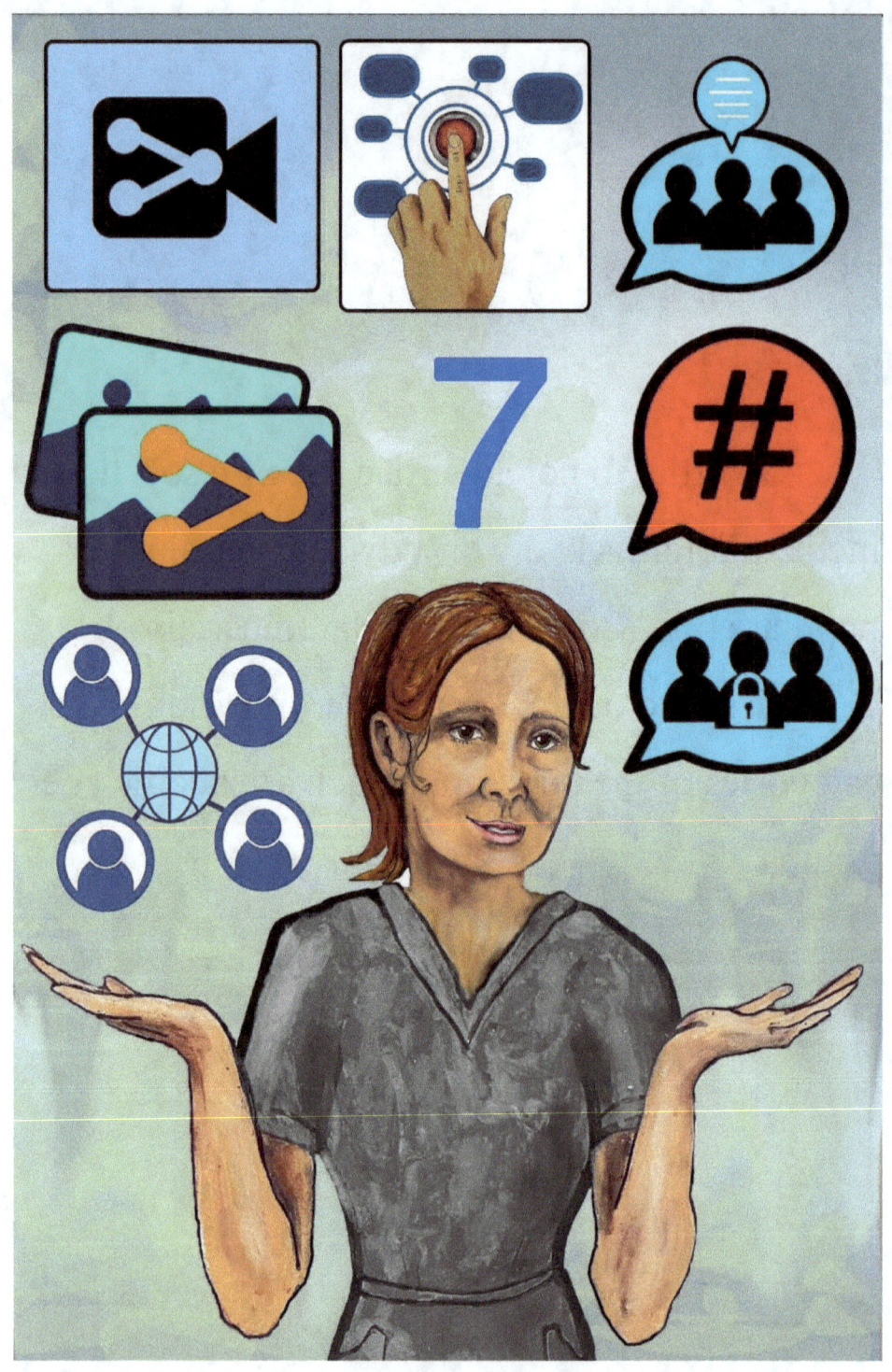

"Social media can be classified into 7 different types. They are social networking, photo sharing, video sharing, interactive media, blogging and community building, microblogging, and private community."

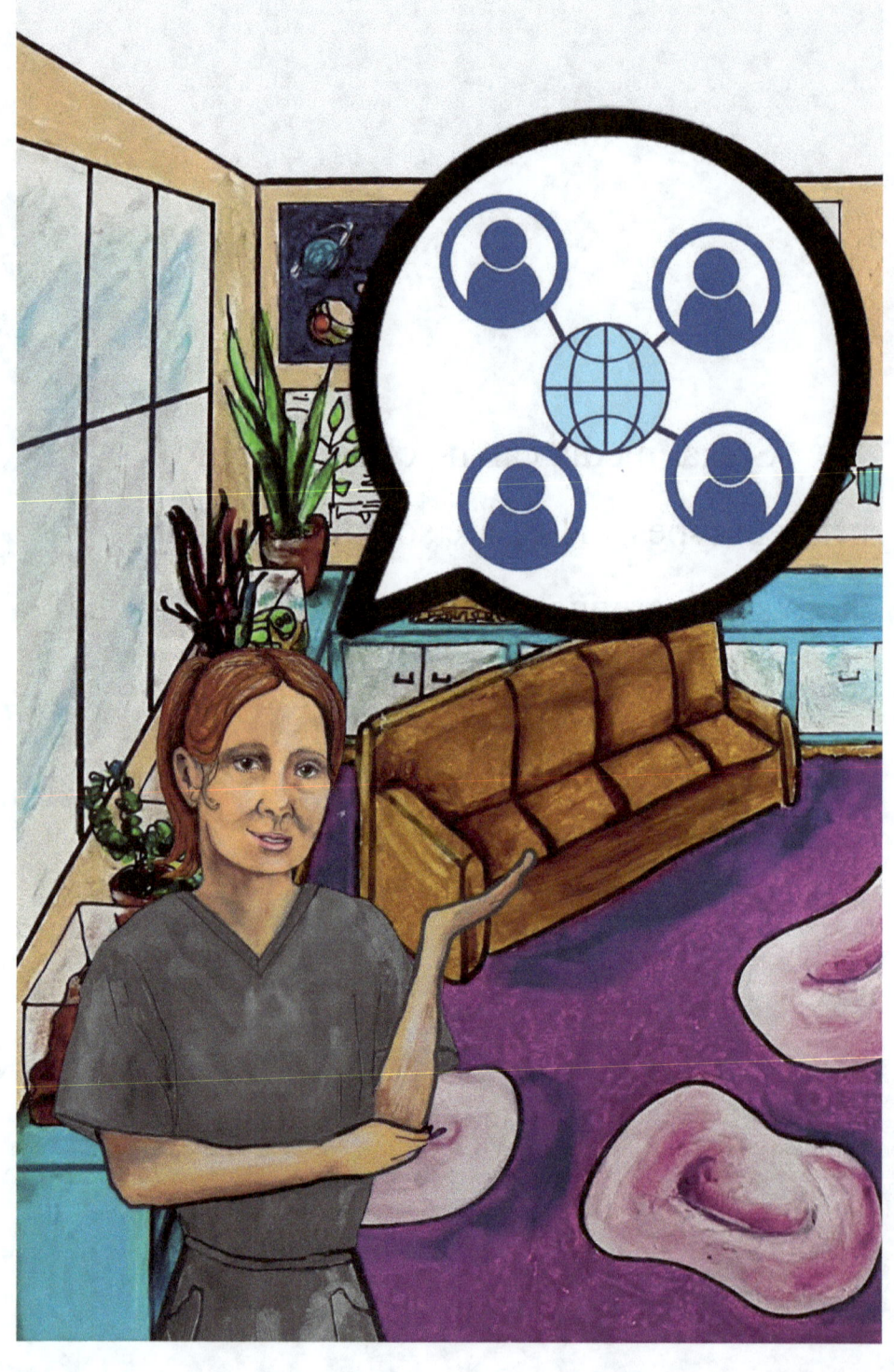

"The first type is social networking. Many social media platforms can be grouped into this type. These social networking sites might integrate scheduling tools so you can organize things and can share photos and videos."

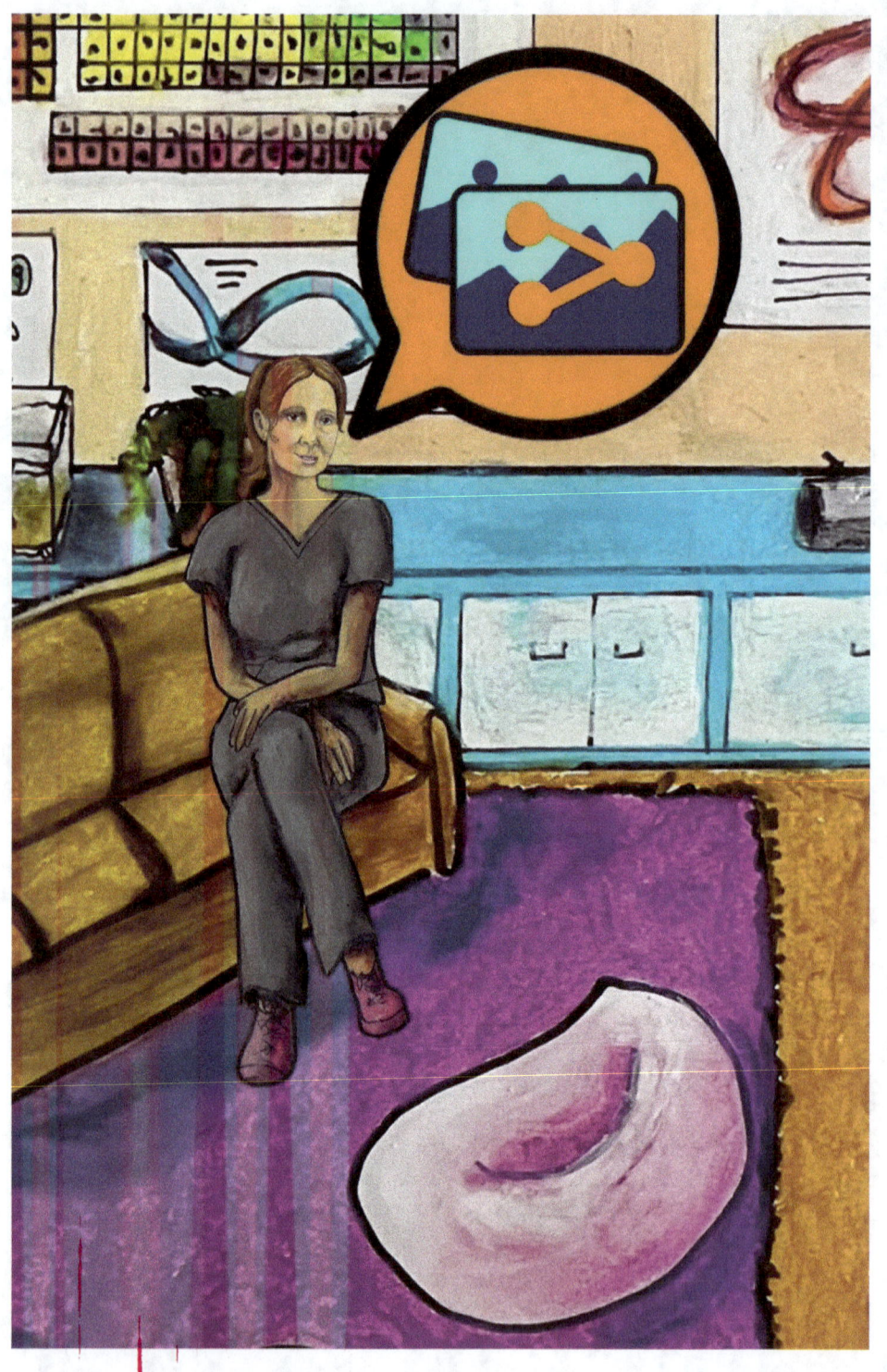

"The second type of social media is photo sharing. The main purpose is self-explanatory."

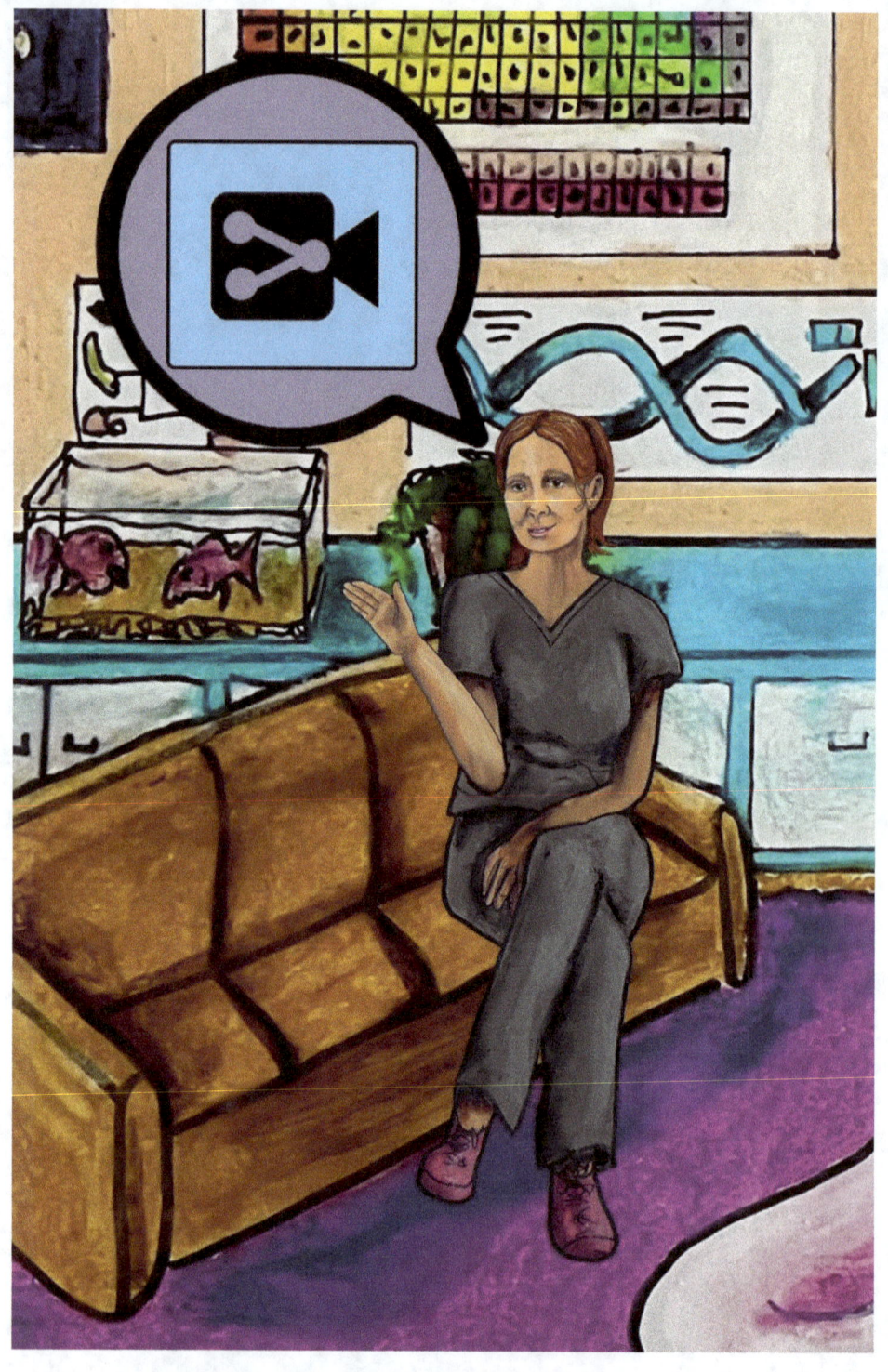

"The third type is video sharing. As the name implies, this type focuses on sharing videos with others."

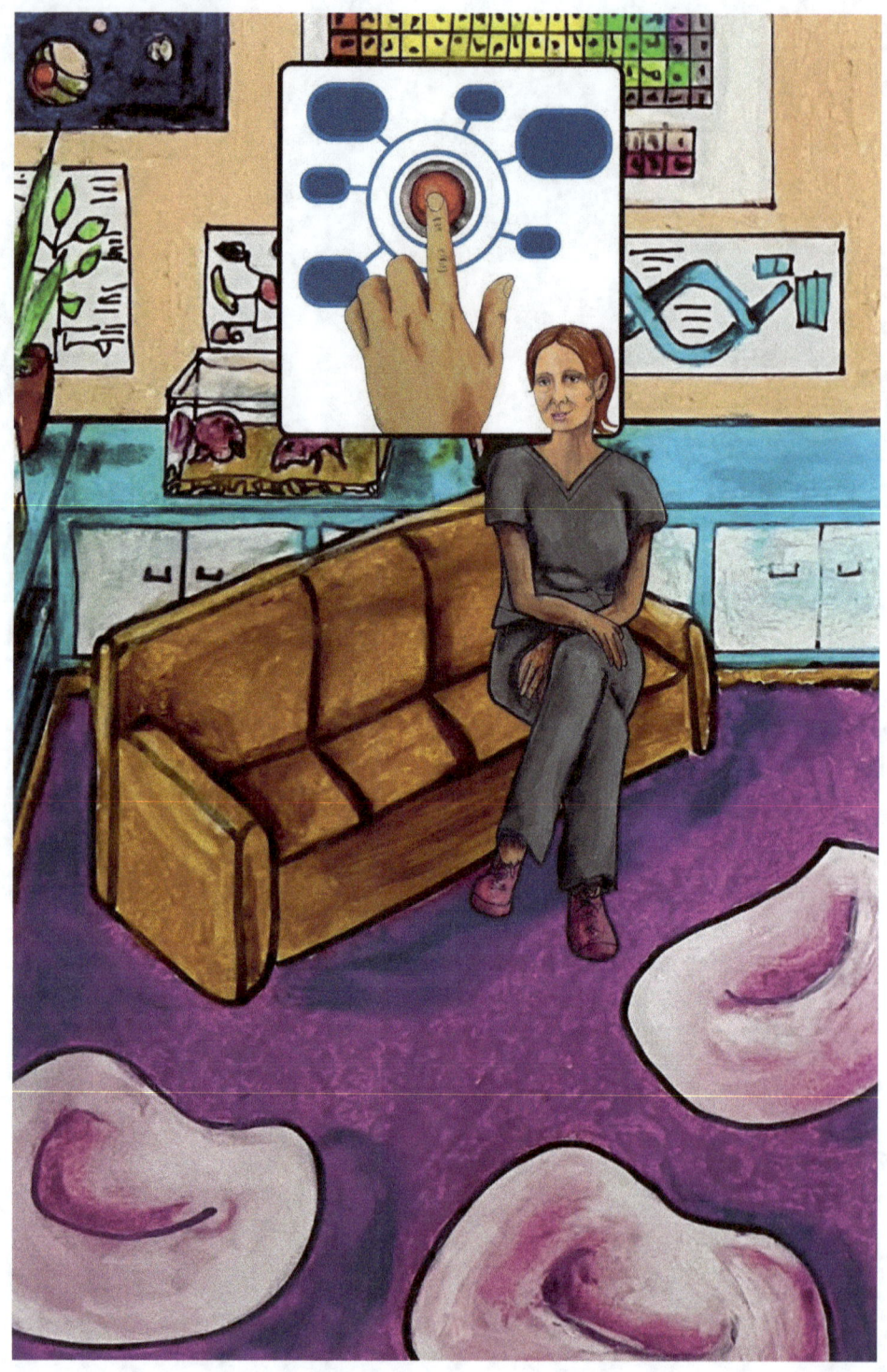

"The fourth type of social media is interactive media. These let users share photos and videos with visual filters and music overlays. In some instances, they may include interactive games."

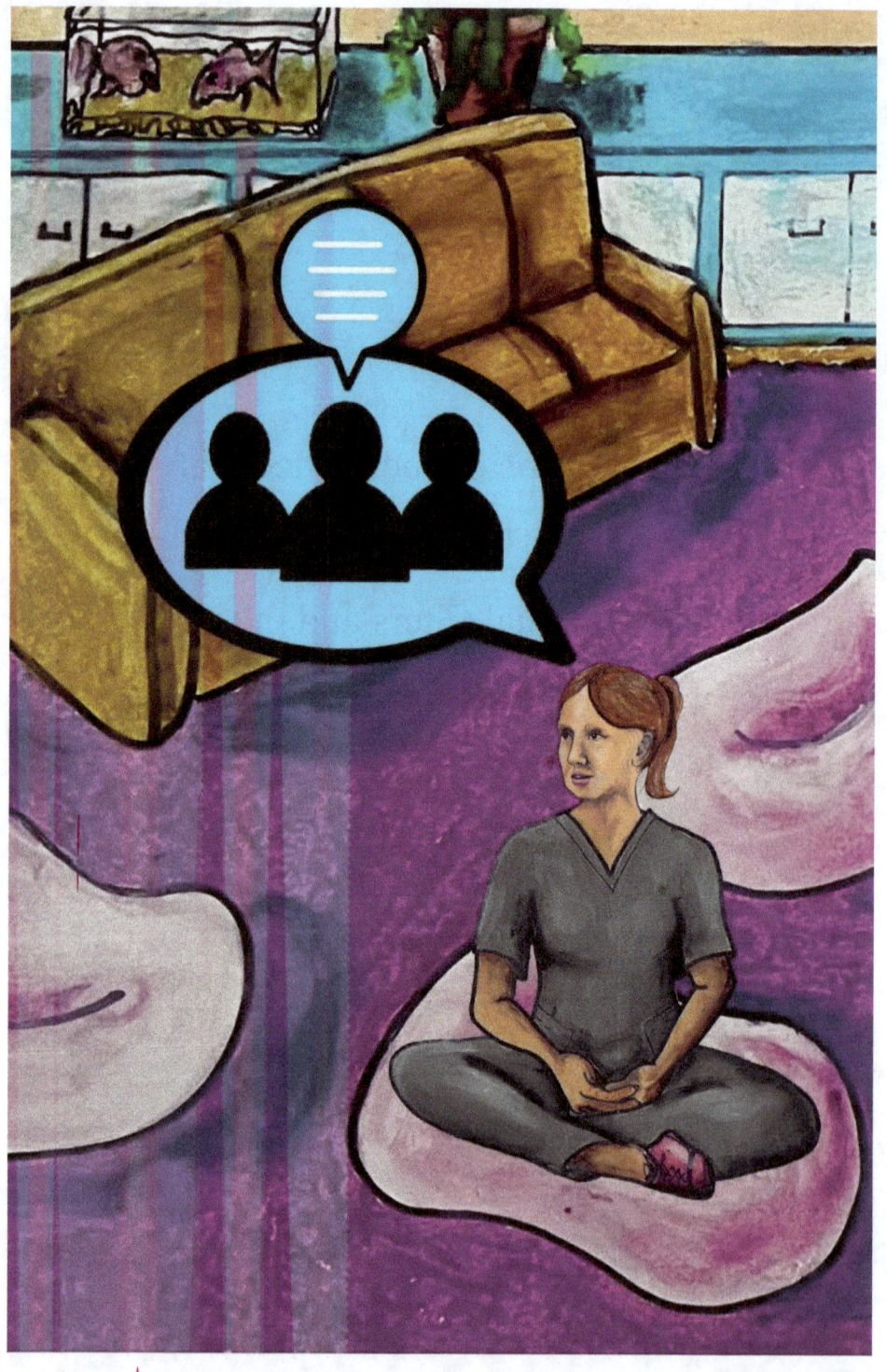

"The fifth type is blogging and community building. This type allows users to share their opinions about topics, events, culture, and various other categories."

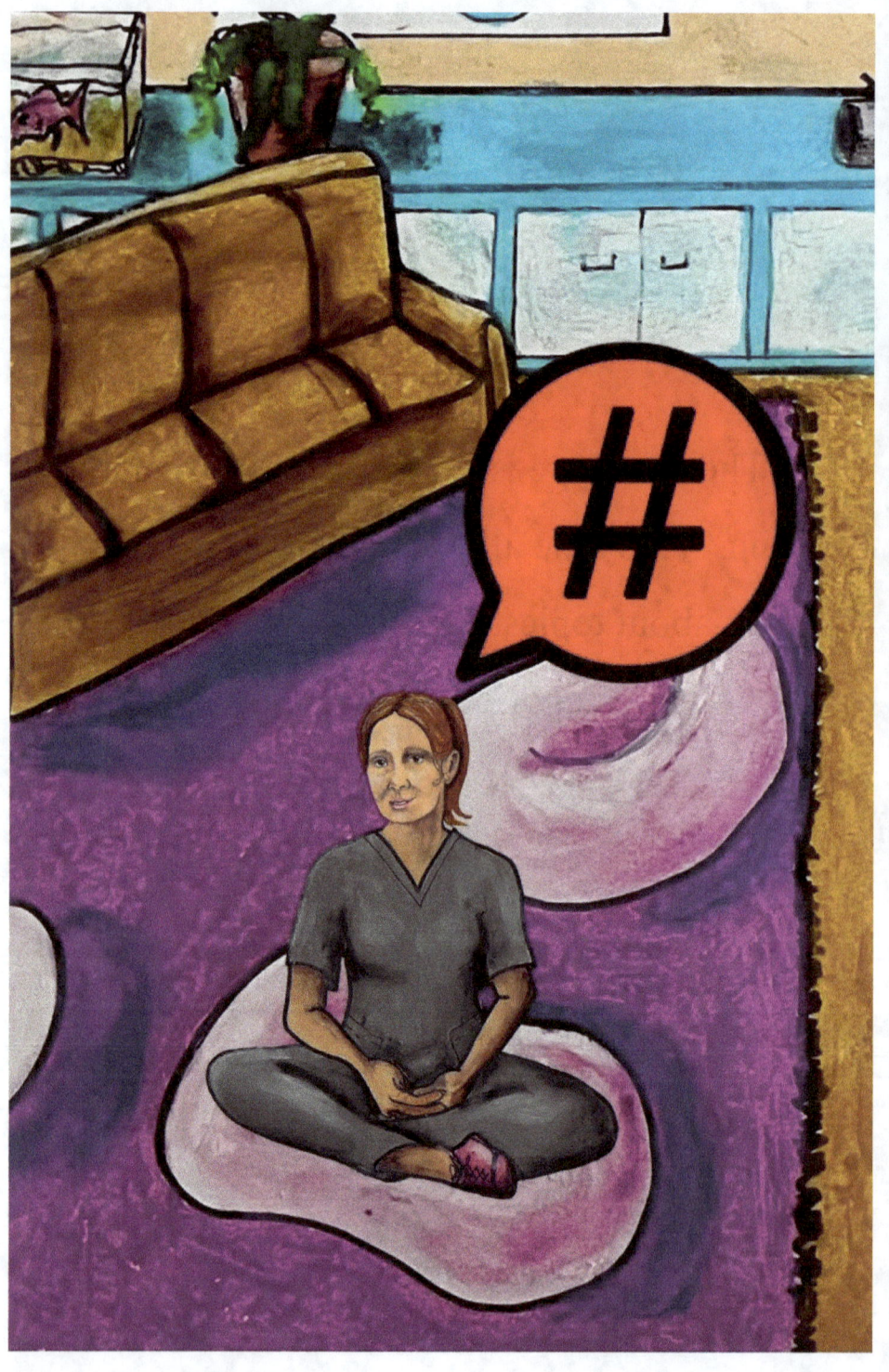

"The sixth type of social media is micro-blogging. This allows users to post very short remarks for others to quickly read and respond."

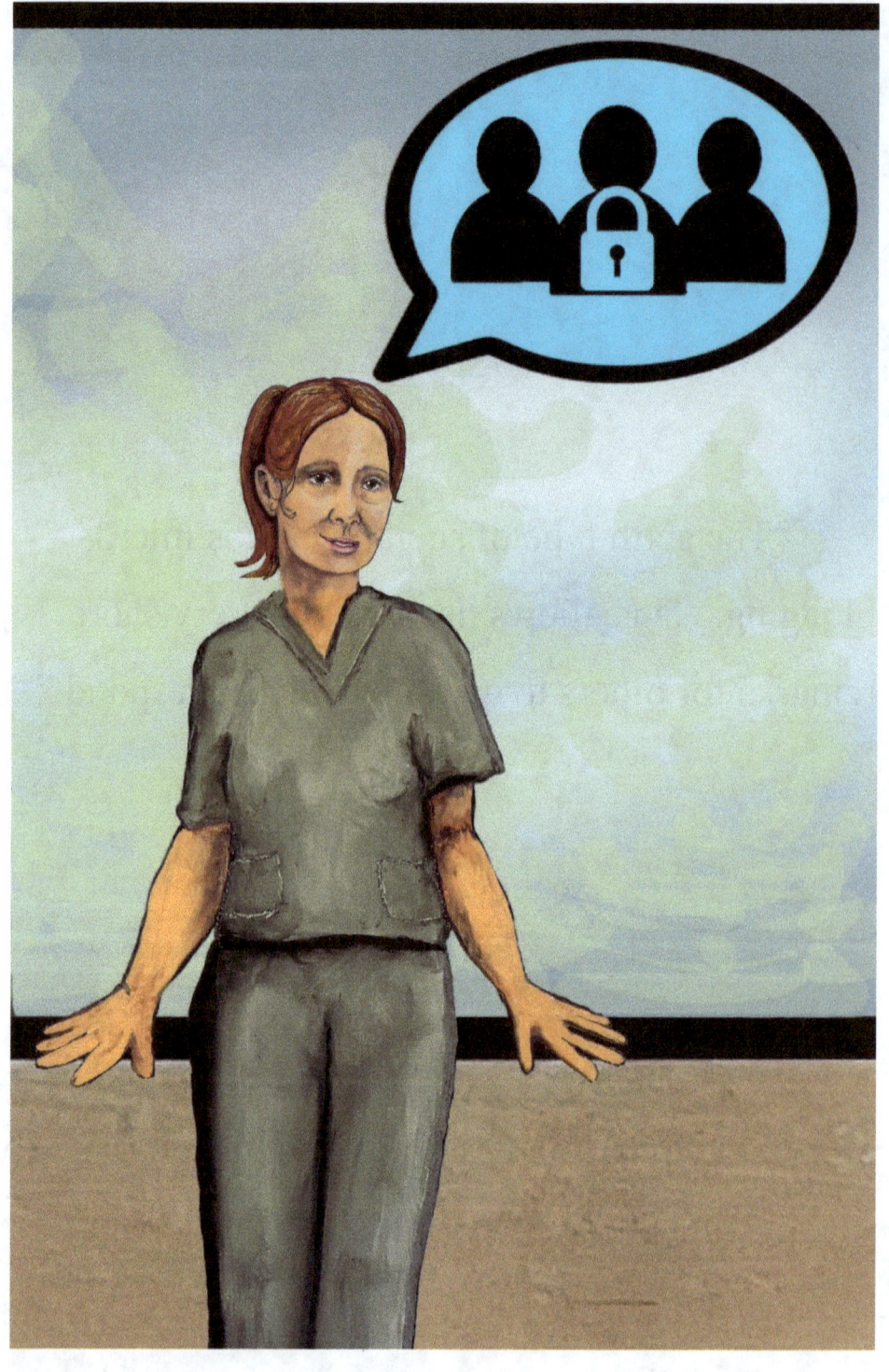

"The last type of social media is called private community. This allows users to talk to each other about very specific topics for which you may not want to go outside of your target audience."

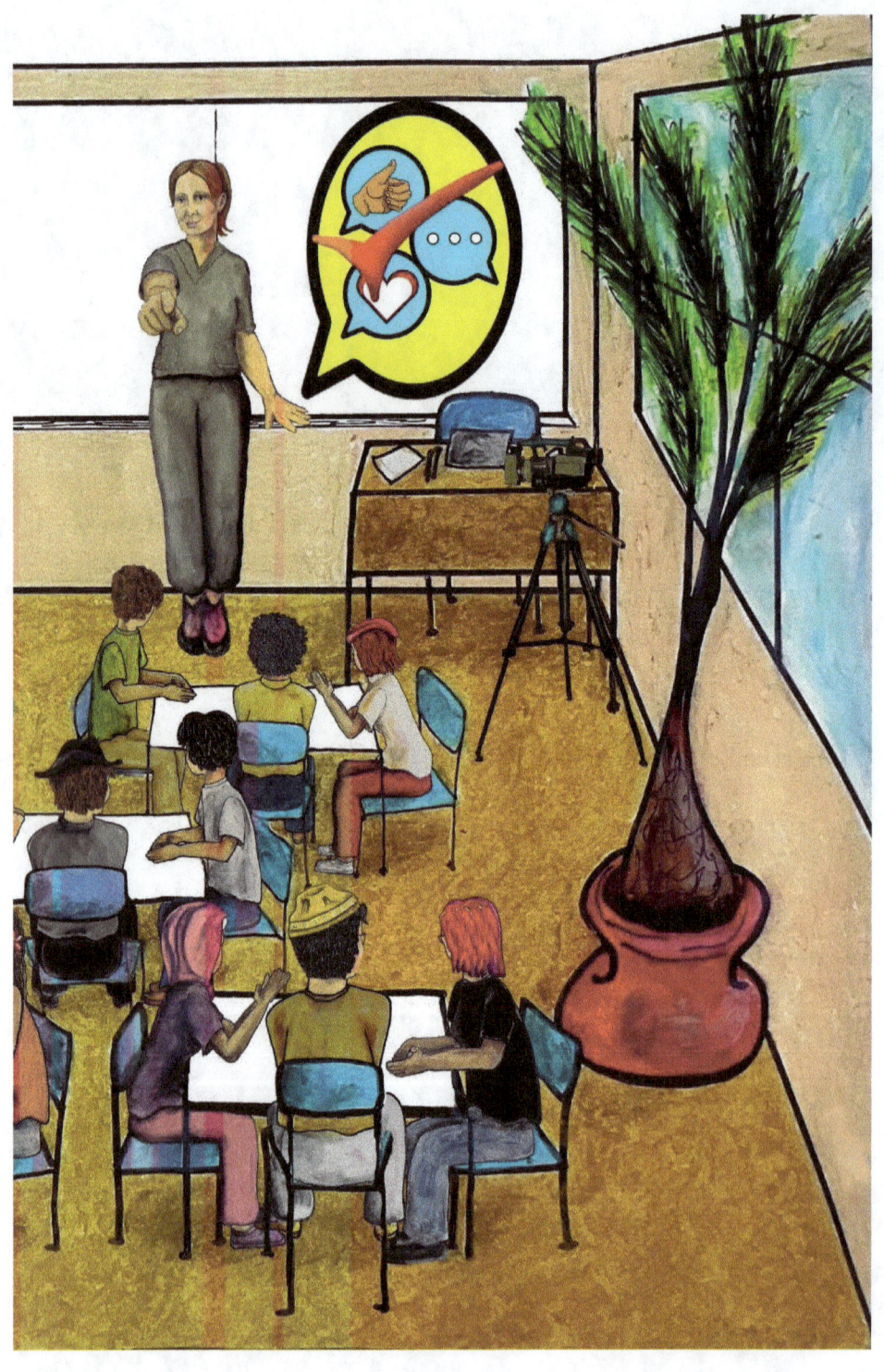

"Now, I would like all of you in the room, those watching the show, and those reading the book, to think about your experiences with social media and share the positive things you have gotten from using it. Share with those around you or write in your journal. Please take the time to do that now."

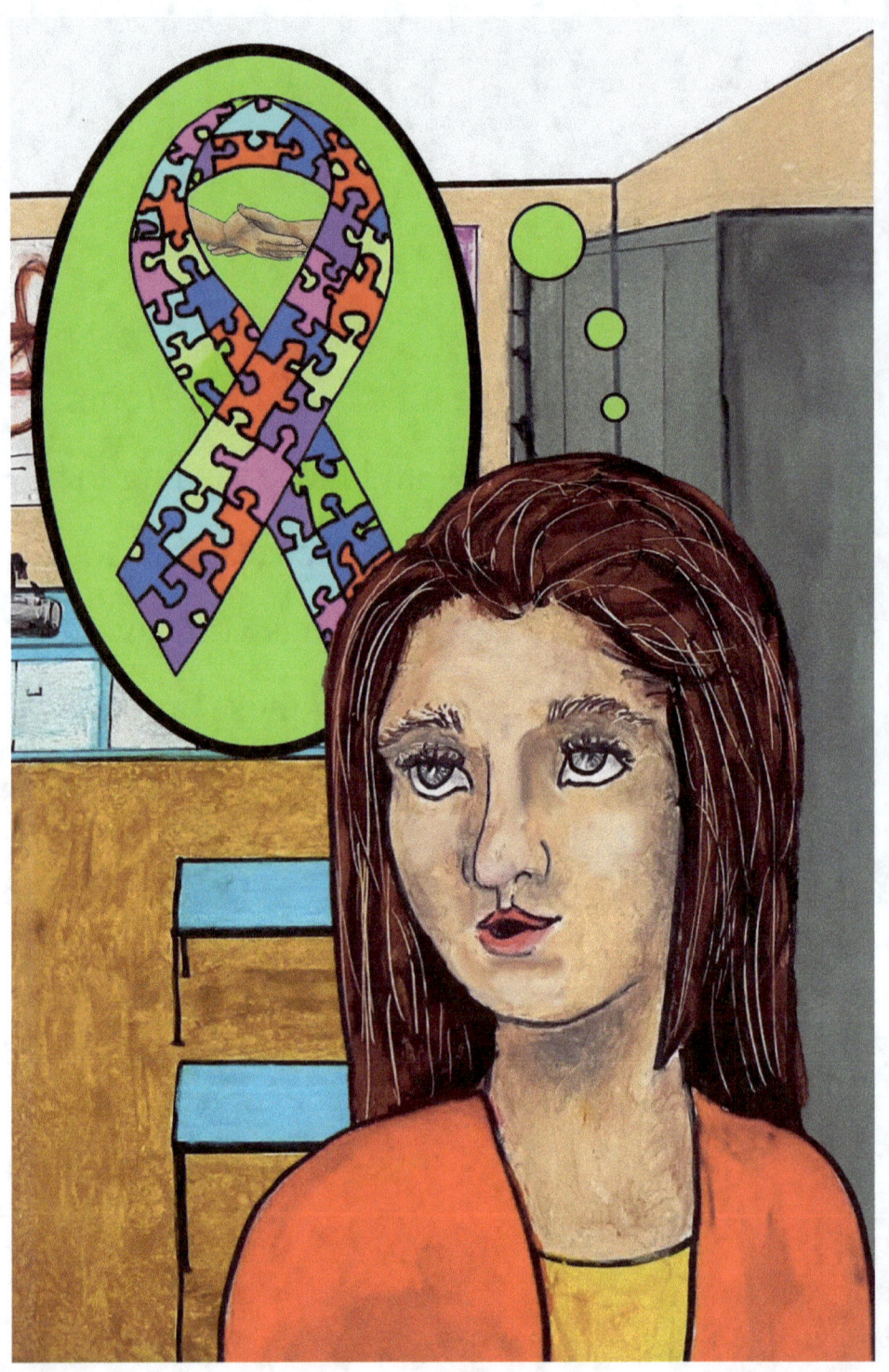

Awira raises her hand, and Nurse Dorothea calls on her to talk. "If you have impaired social functioning like being on the autism spectrum, social media can provide an outlet to help communicate with others and share your thoughts in a safe space. Also, if you are a shy person and don't like speaking up, social media can help a person share their opinion when they otherwise would not."

"You're definitely right that social media can help people with disabilities," says Nurse Dorothea.

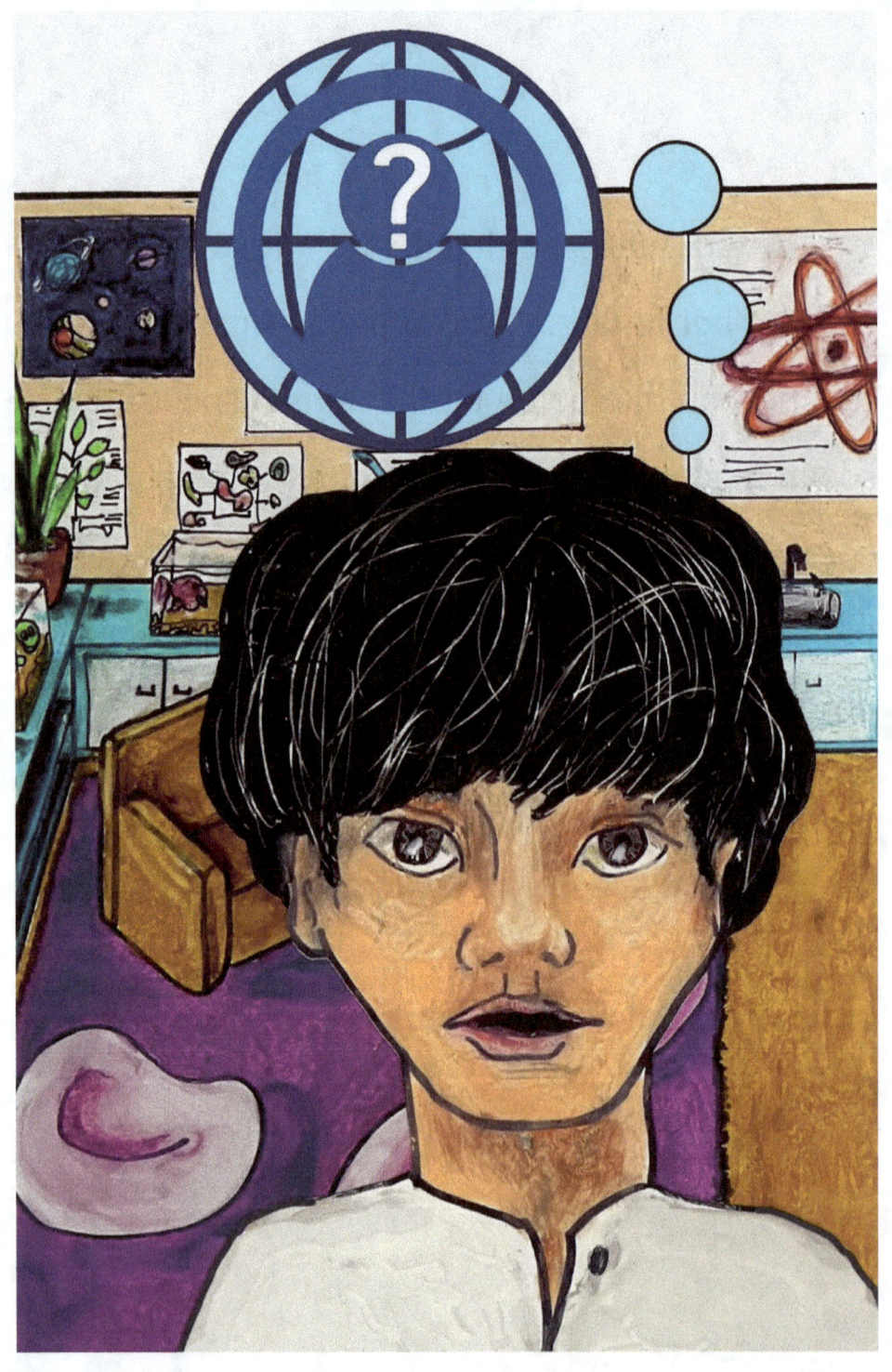

Antonio raises his hand, and Nurse Dorothea calls on him to talk. "If you are in a stigmatized group, like having a mental illness, and people may be quick to judge you as wrong or bad, then having anonymity in social media while still sharing your opinions about things is very helpful."

"Good point. Pope Francis said the thing he missed most once becoming Pope was anonymity. Being unknown and still doing basic human things can be very important," says Nurse Dorothea.

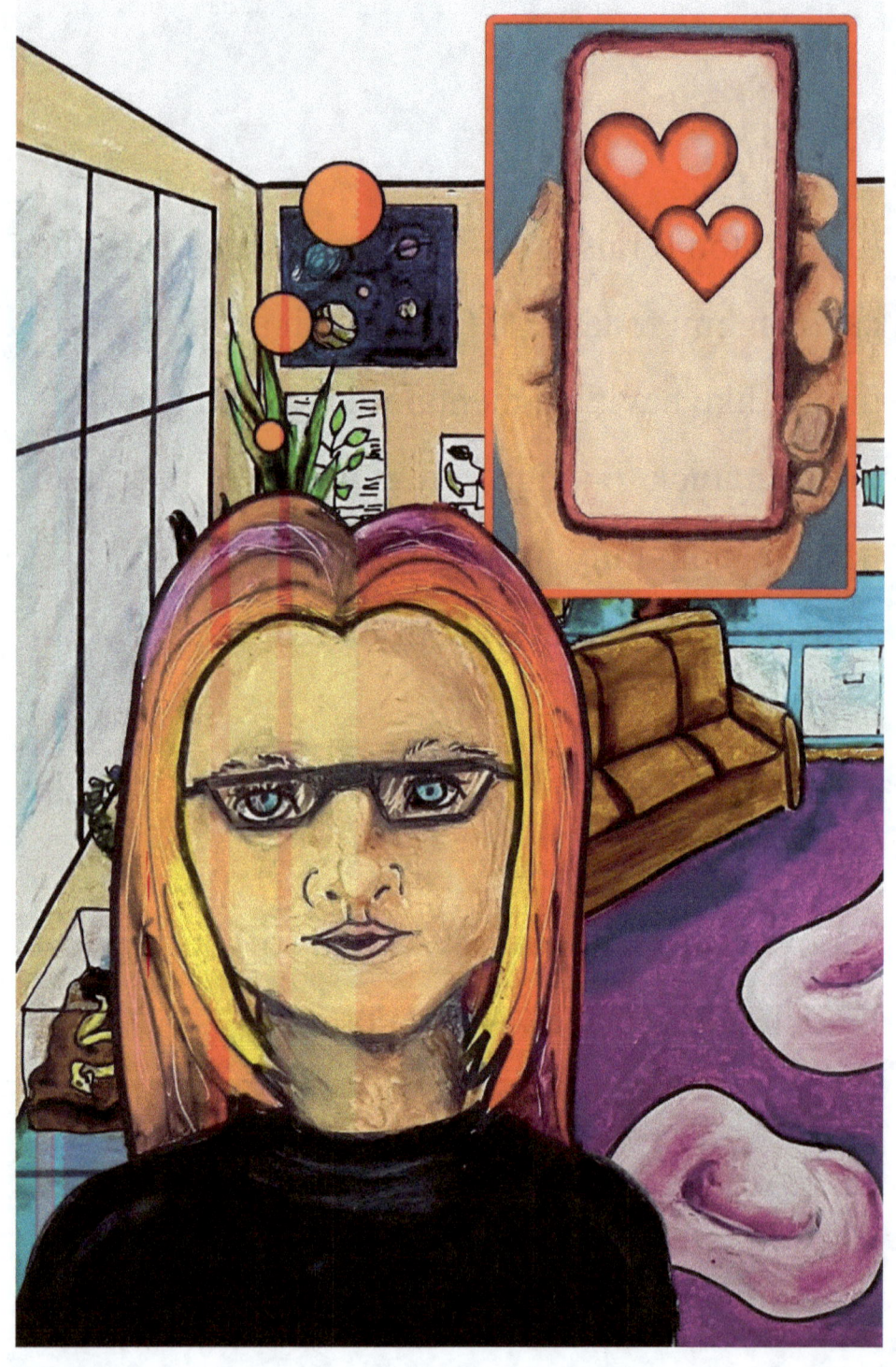

Juniper raises her hand, and Nurse Dorothea calls on her to talk. "It can be easy to form friendships online if you have an illness and cannot leave the home. We all need friends and people to communicate with, and social media gives an opportunity for some people who would not have that option."

"Excellent," says Nurse Dorothea.

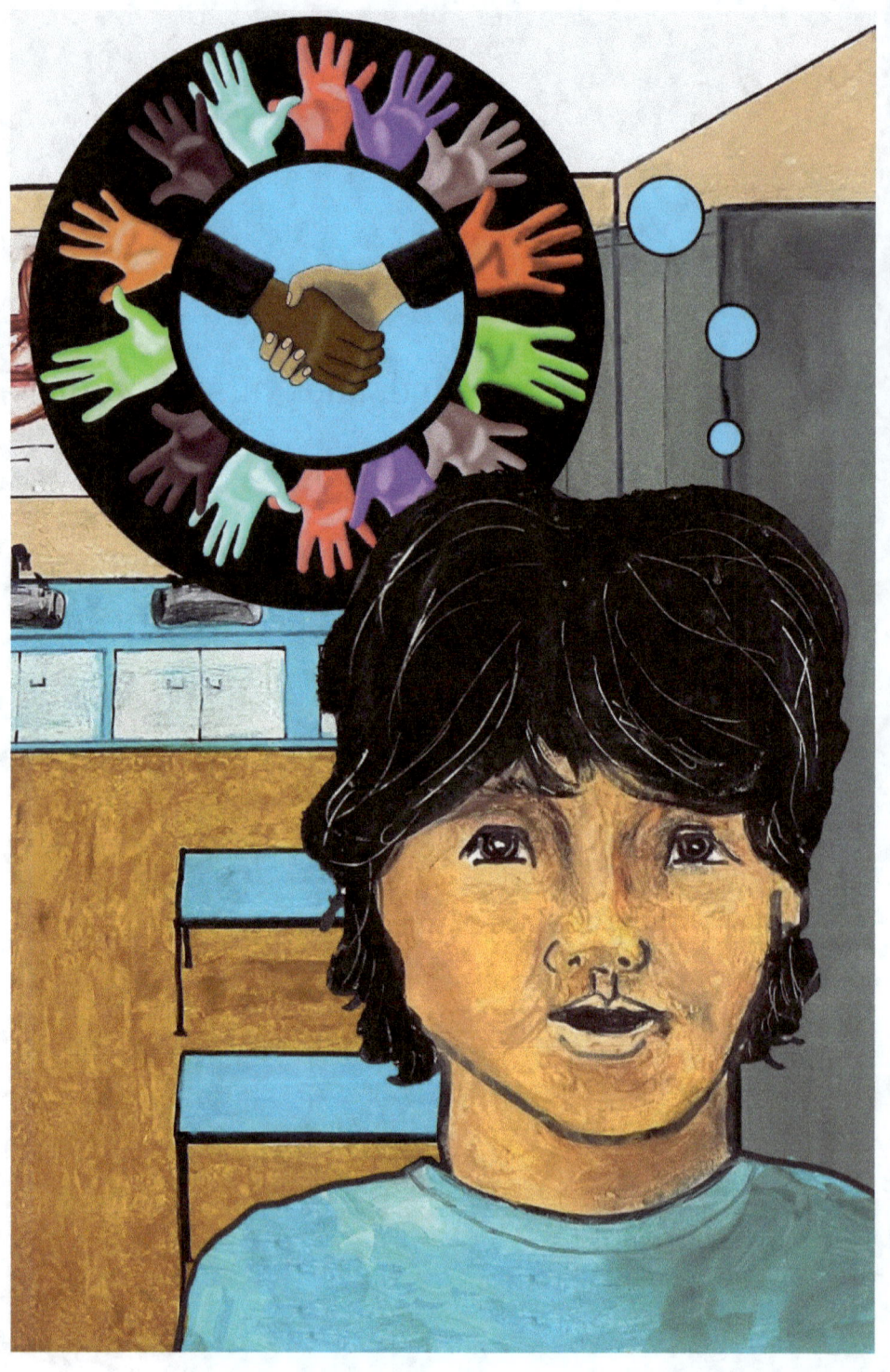

Ji Ho raises his hand, and Nurse Dorothea calls on him to talk. "I think social media can be good because it can encourage community engagement so that people of different races, ethnicities, cultures, and backgrounds can interact with each other in a safe environment when they may not interact in the non-digital world."

"We are only getting to the future together, so learning to talk with each other in a safe place will help our transition to the future be smoother," says Nurse Dorothea.

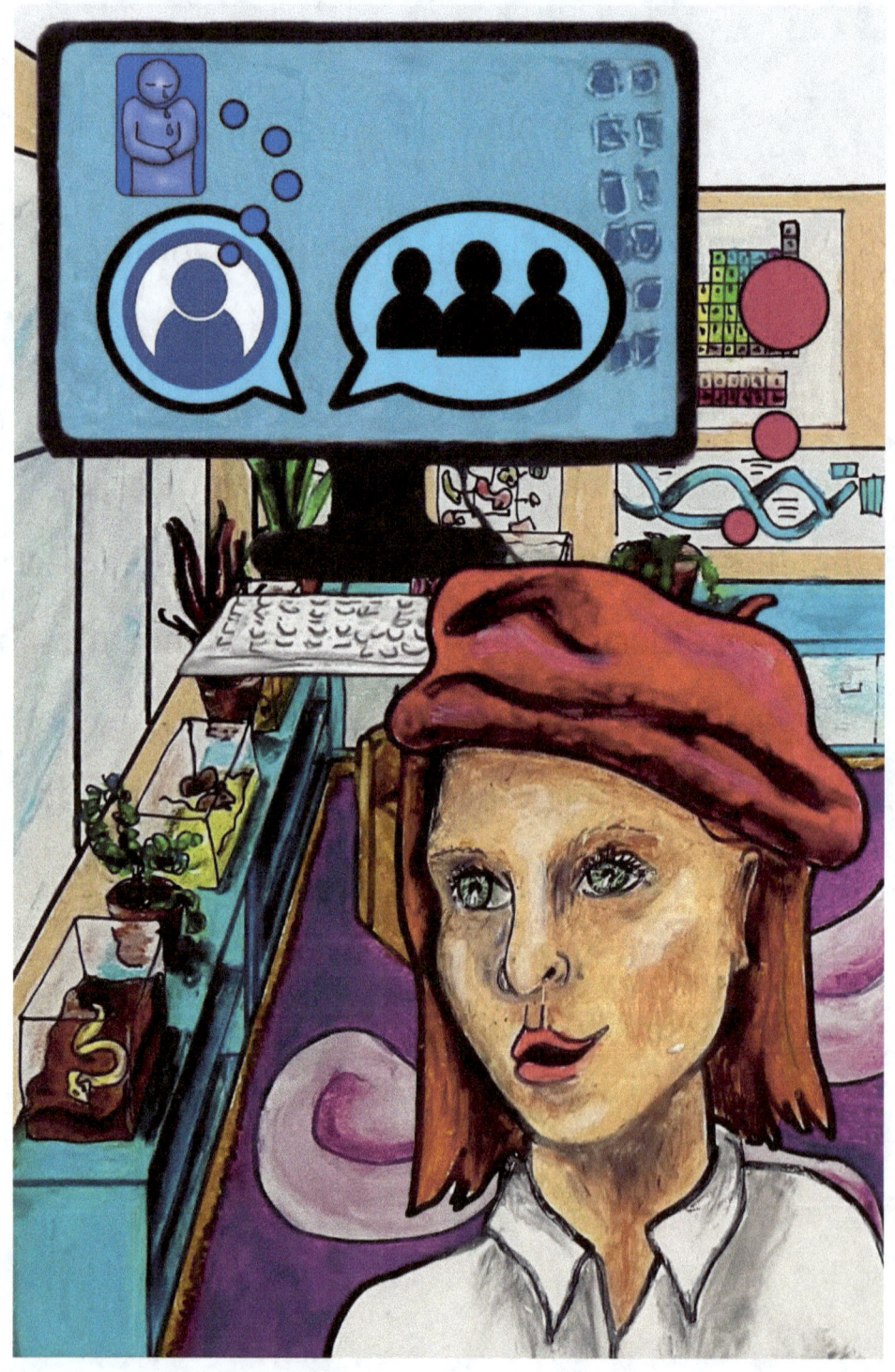

Maria raises her hand, and Nurse Dorothea calls on her to talk. "If you are depressed, it is sometimes much easier to talk with other people. You can determine when and how much you want to talk to someone. Maybe in certain times of the day, it is better to interact with others so having that choice when to interact can be very important."

"Great thought. The digital world allows us to choose when we want to interact with others, which can give people with depressed moods options to express their emotions," says Nurse Dorothea.

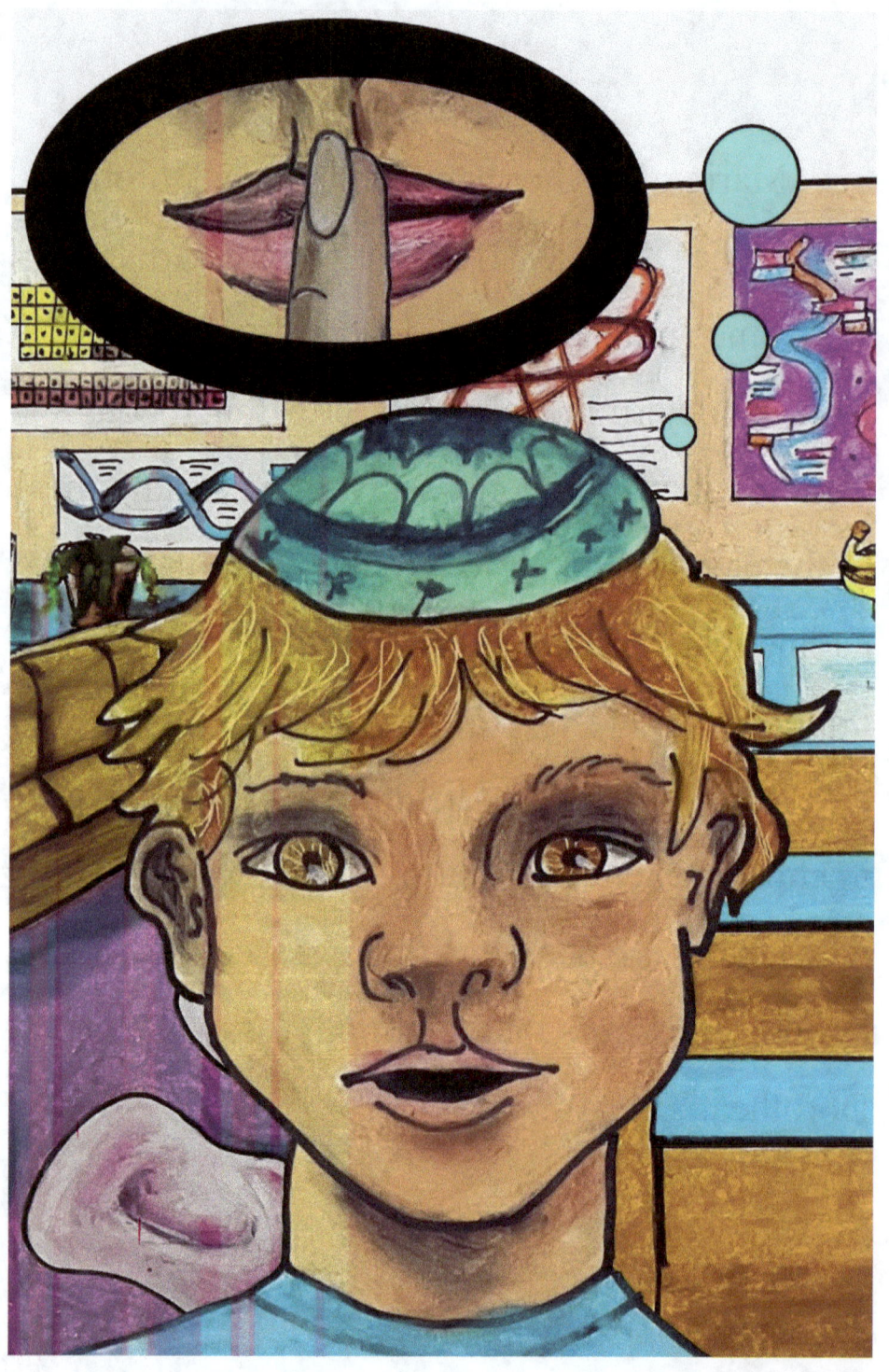

Levi raises his hand, and Nurse Dorothea calls on him to talk. "Digital conversations do not require non-verbal cues of when and what to talk about, so for those of us who struggle with learning body language, the digital world provides an easier space to communicate. For example, sometimes in the past, I would get too physically close to someone when I talked with them, and they would get annoyed. I don't have to worry about that in the digital world."

"Non-verbal cues have to be learned, and you're right that some people have a hard time learning them," says Nurse Dorothea.

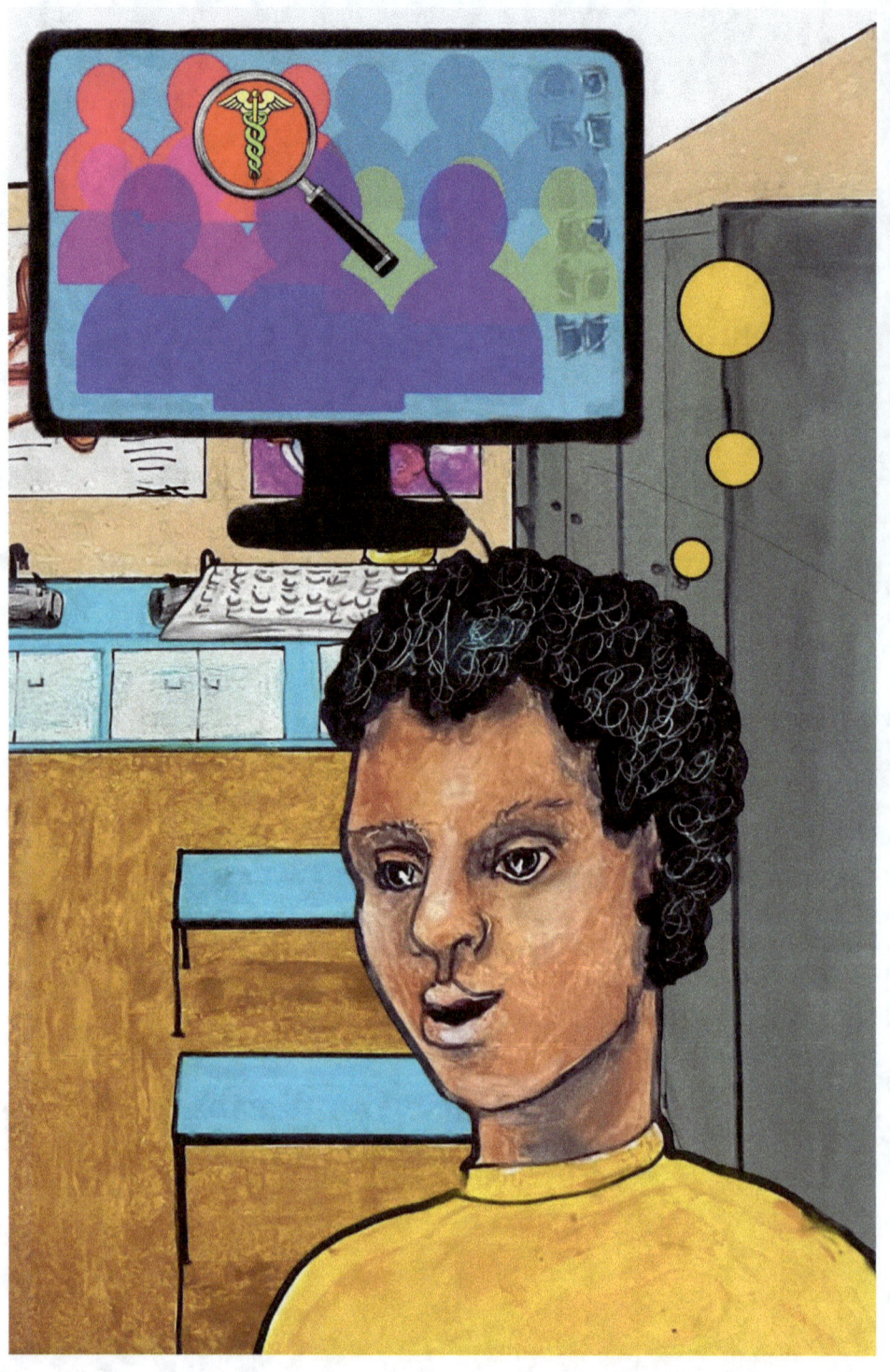

Ekon raises his hand, and Nurse Dorothea calls on him to talk. "Having an online support group regarding an ADHD diagnosis has been helpful. We share info about the illness, discuss symptoms, and how medications help us."

"Support groups are very helpful, and I'm glad you've found one that works for you," says Nurse Dorothea.

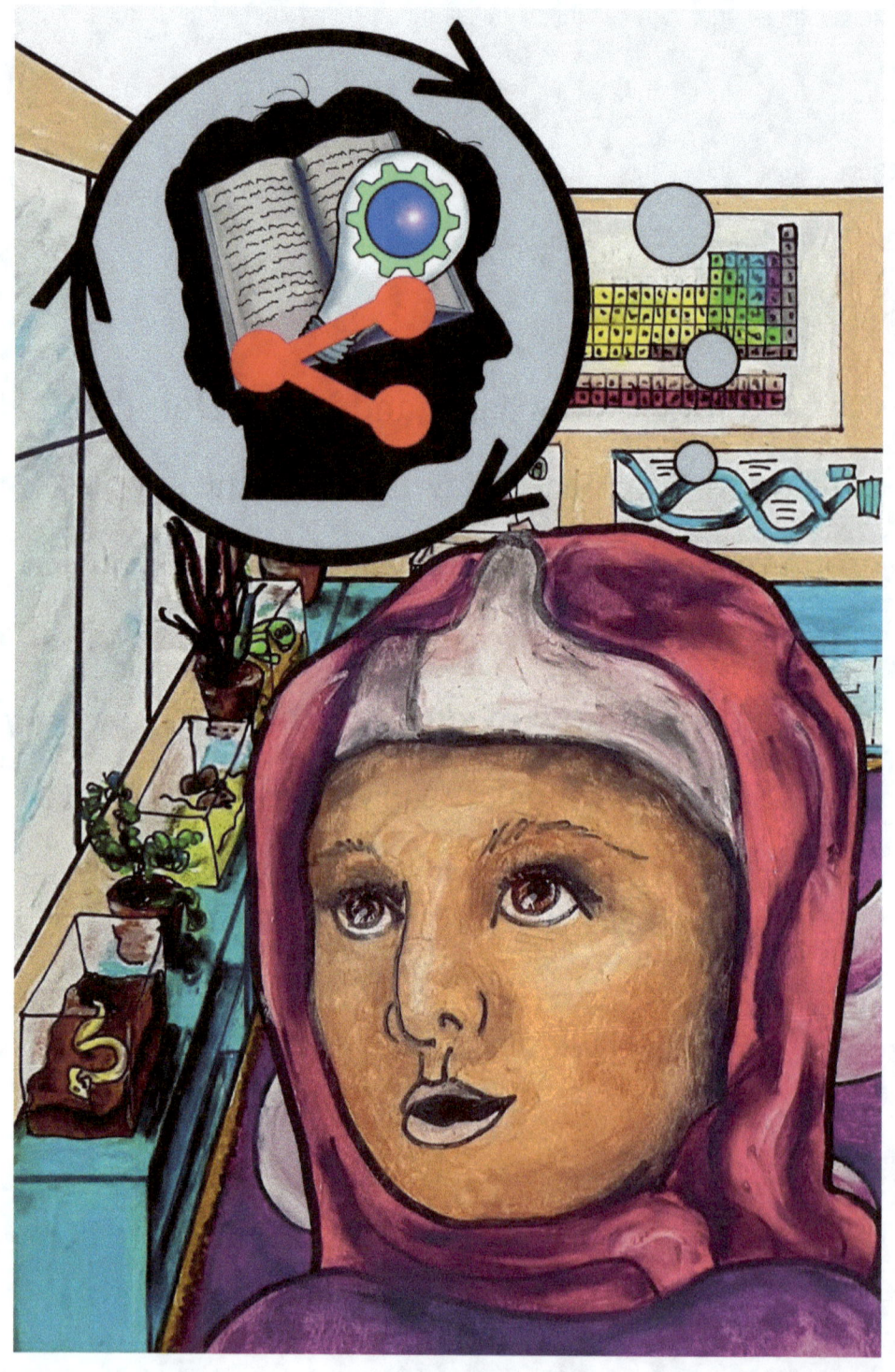

Fatima raises her hand, and Nurse Dorothea calls on her to talk. "I think social media makes it easier to share experiences with others. You can do it with just pictures, a short video of something fun you have done, or a short sentence post about something you liked."

"Sharing our human experience with others is important and helps us create a culture we want to be in and contribute to," says Nurse Dorothea.

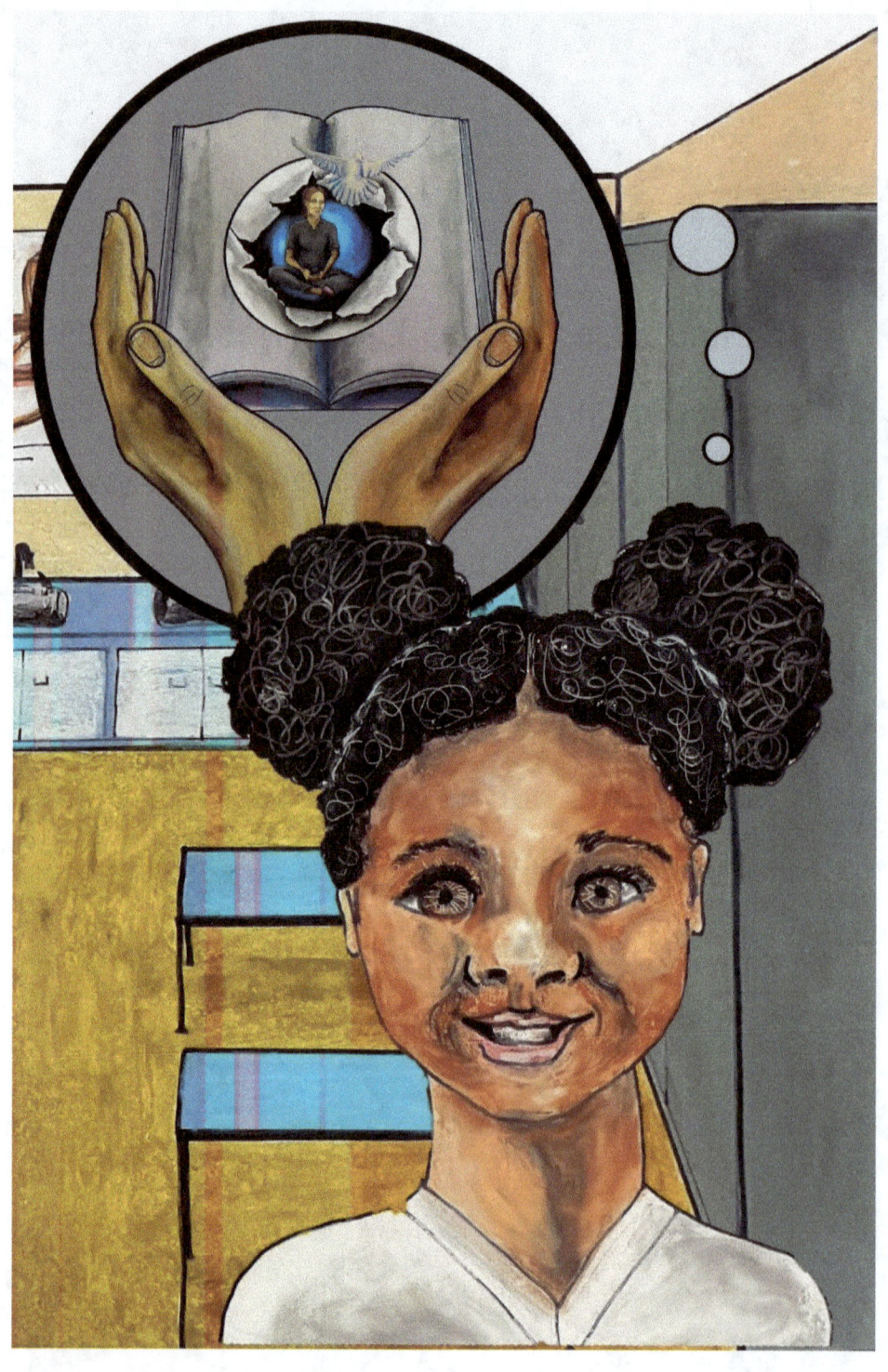

Amisha raises her hand, and Nurse Dorothea calls on her to talk. "Getting tips from my friends online about coping skills that can be useful for different situations has been very helpful in my life. I don't think I would be where I am today if it weren't for the tips I've received from all my friends."

"There are so many different coping skills that having a community where you can share your ideas with others is great," says Nurse Dorothea.

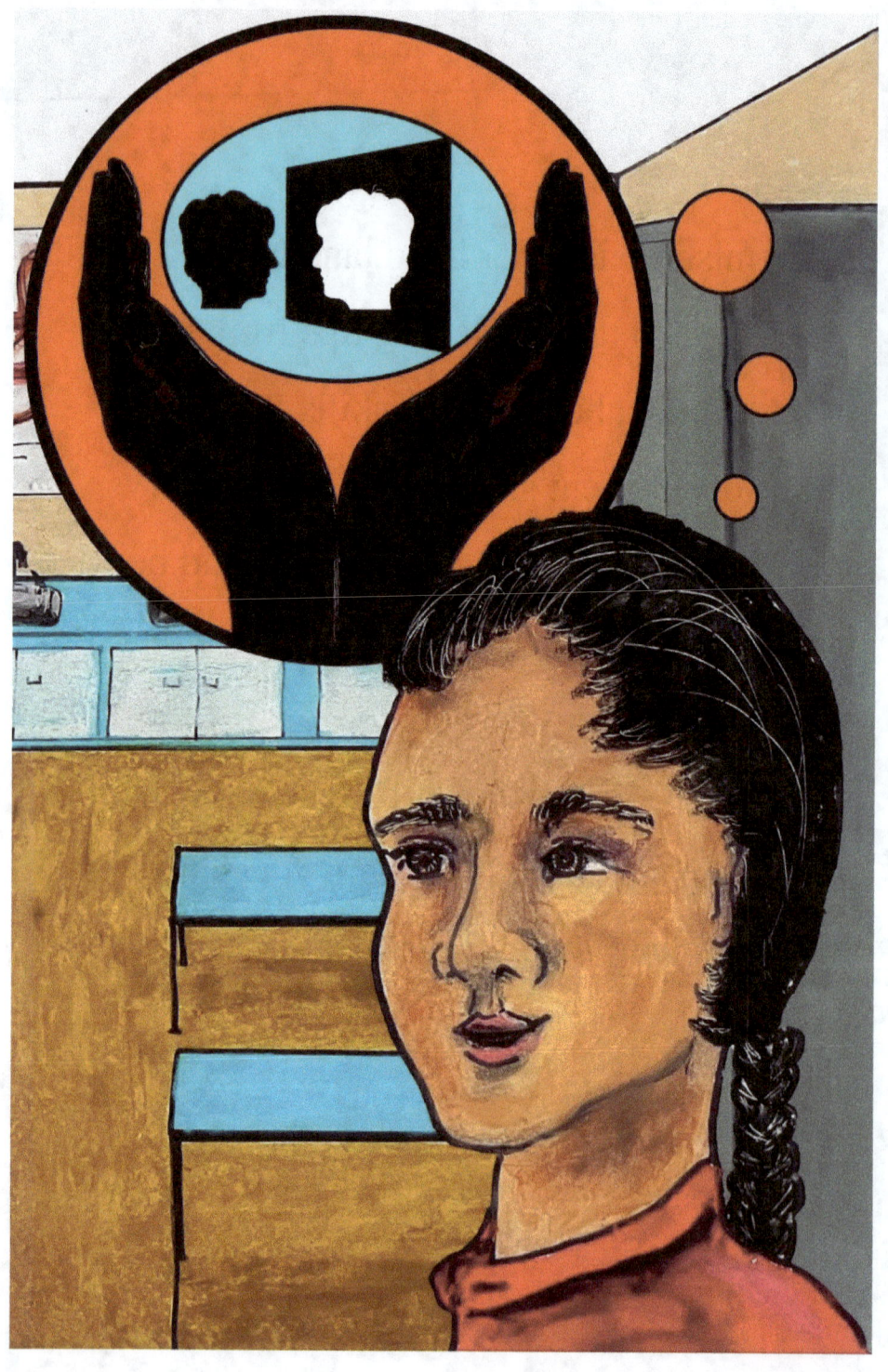

Pia raises her hand, and Nurse Dorothea calls on her to talk. "I think social media has helped me with self-disclosure. I've learned to do it gradually and not share my whole life story with every person I meet. Self-disclosure should be a give and take. What I mean is that if someone discloses a little something about themselves, then you should do the same and disclose at least the same amount. It's fun to learn about others, but I think we should do it gradually over time."

"Great point. We should always be careful what we are disclosing," says Nurse Dorothea.

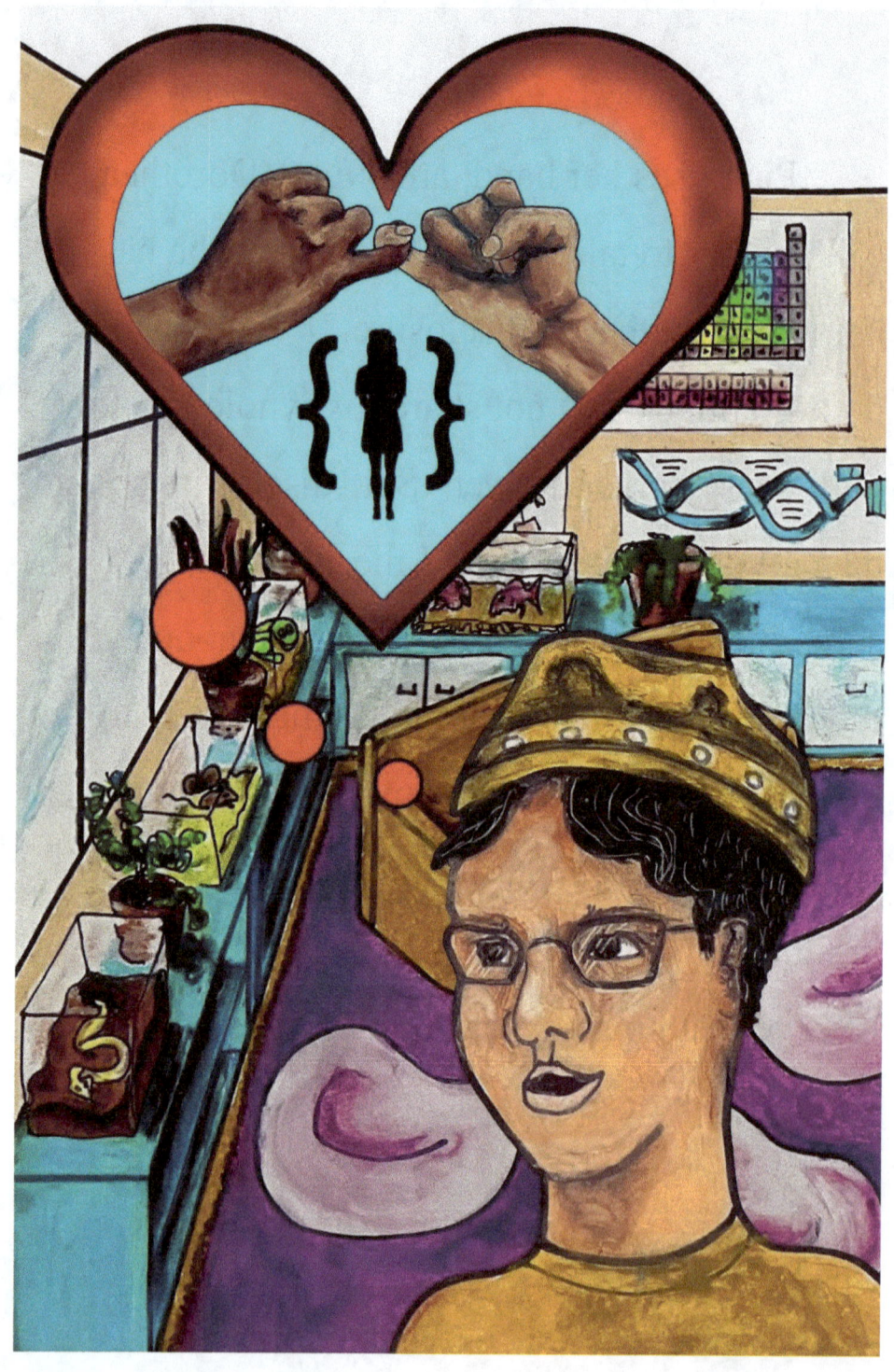

Azamat raises his hand, and Nurse Dorothea calls on him to talk. "Social media has helped me establish new relationships and feel less alone."

"It is very important to form new relationships, but you should use caution when it comes to meeting strangers online since some can pretend to be someone they are not. They may even try to meet you in person and that could be dangerous. Always meet an online friend with others so that you can be safe and tell your parents what you are doing. There are people in the world that create fake online personas which is called catfishing. Be aware of your surroundings, please, since there are predators of the young and the weak in the world," says Nurse Dorothea.

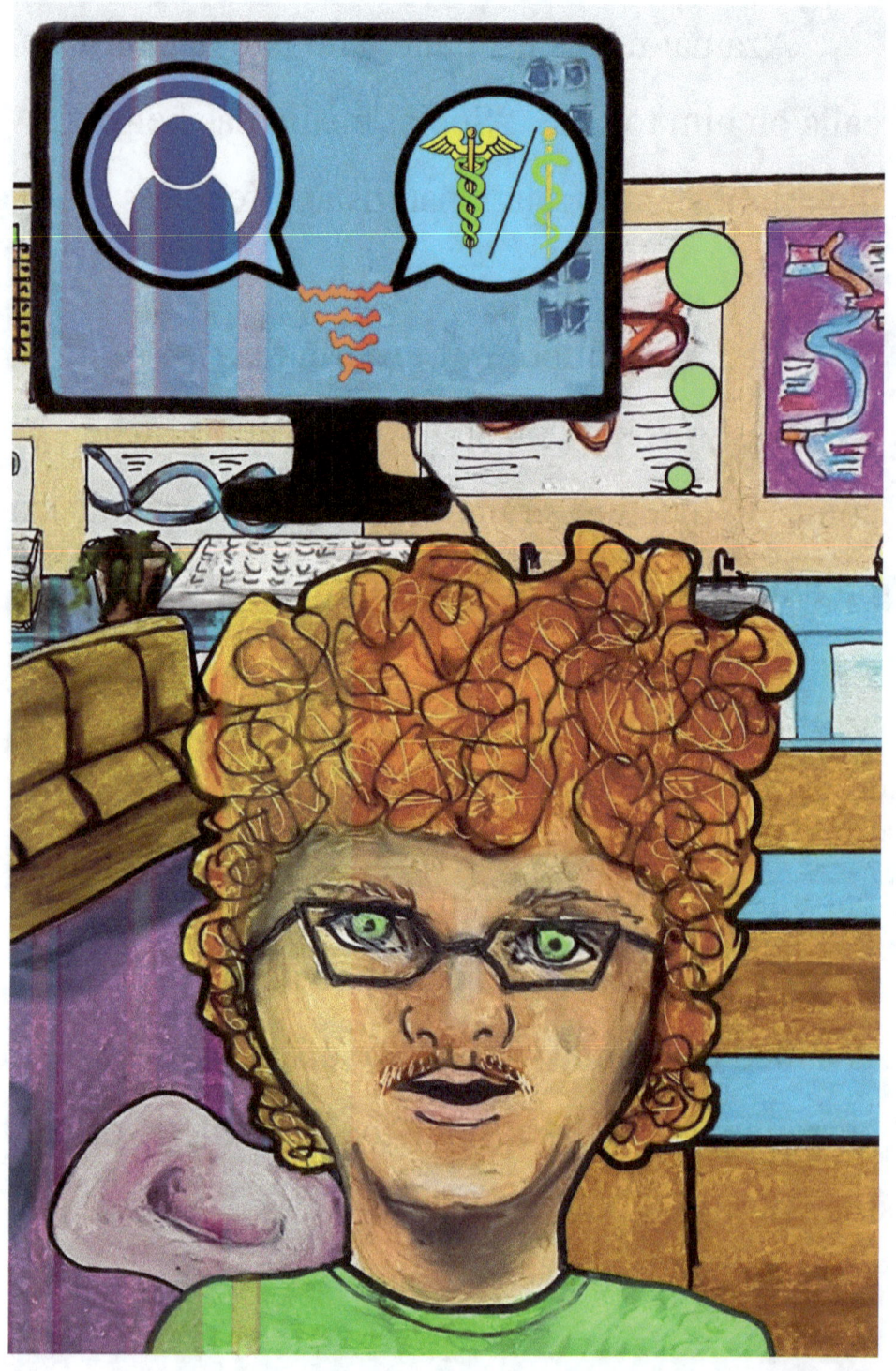

Connor raises his hand, and Nurse Dorothea calls on him to talk. "I think social media has helped me connect with my providers better. I have been able to send emails to my provider to get questions answered quickly instead of having to wait for the next visit which could be months away."

"More and more healthcare providers are starting to use secure emails to talk to patients, and people should use that tool since it can be very effective," says Nurse Dorothea.

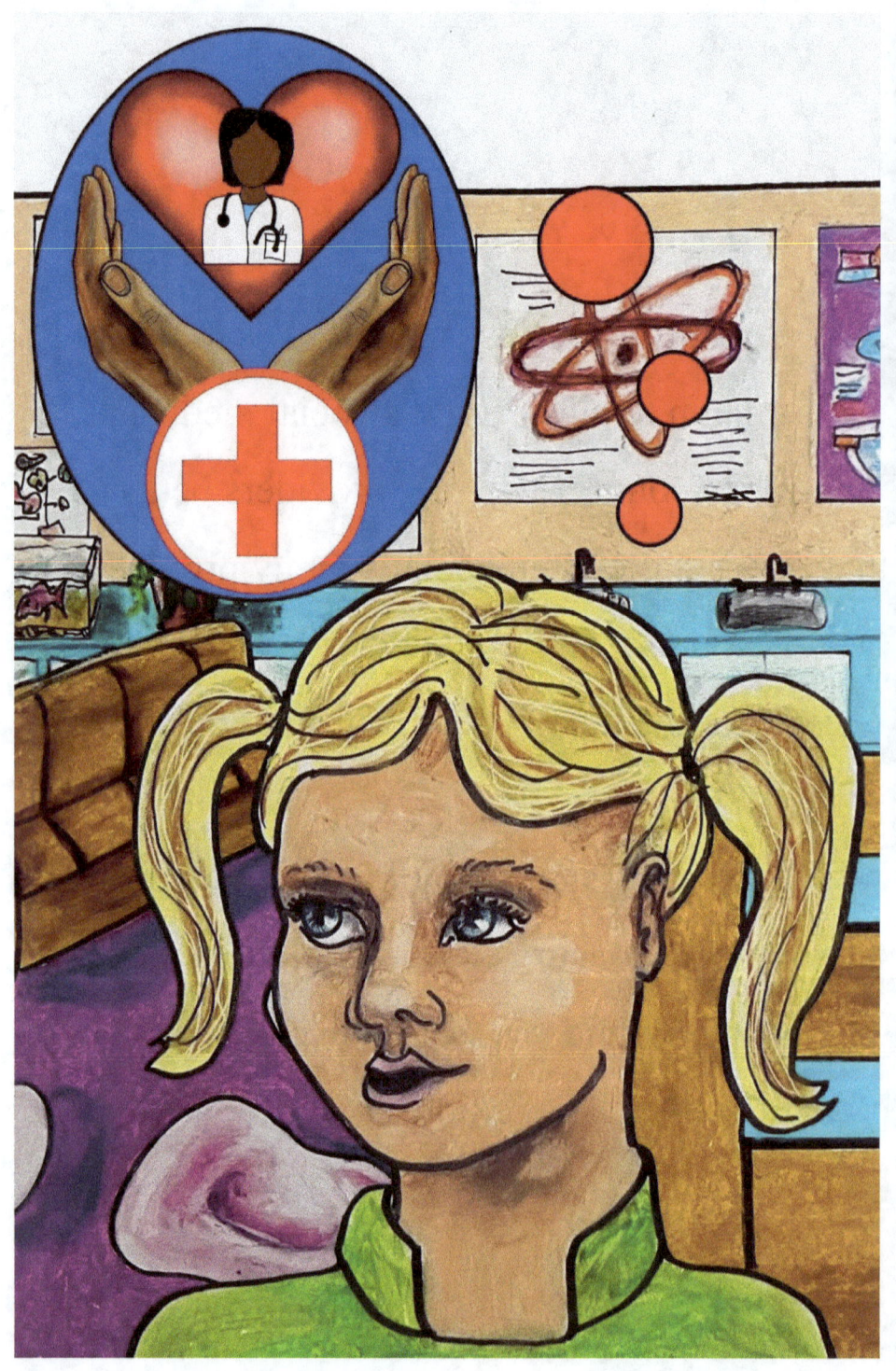

Frida raises her hand, and Nurse Dorothea calls on her to talk. "Social media has helped me have better healthcare. I've gotten information and researched my condition so that when I visit with my Provider, I am better informed and have better questions so that I am more in charge of my own health."

"Knowledge can be power," says Nurse Dorothea.

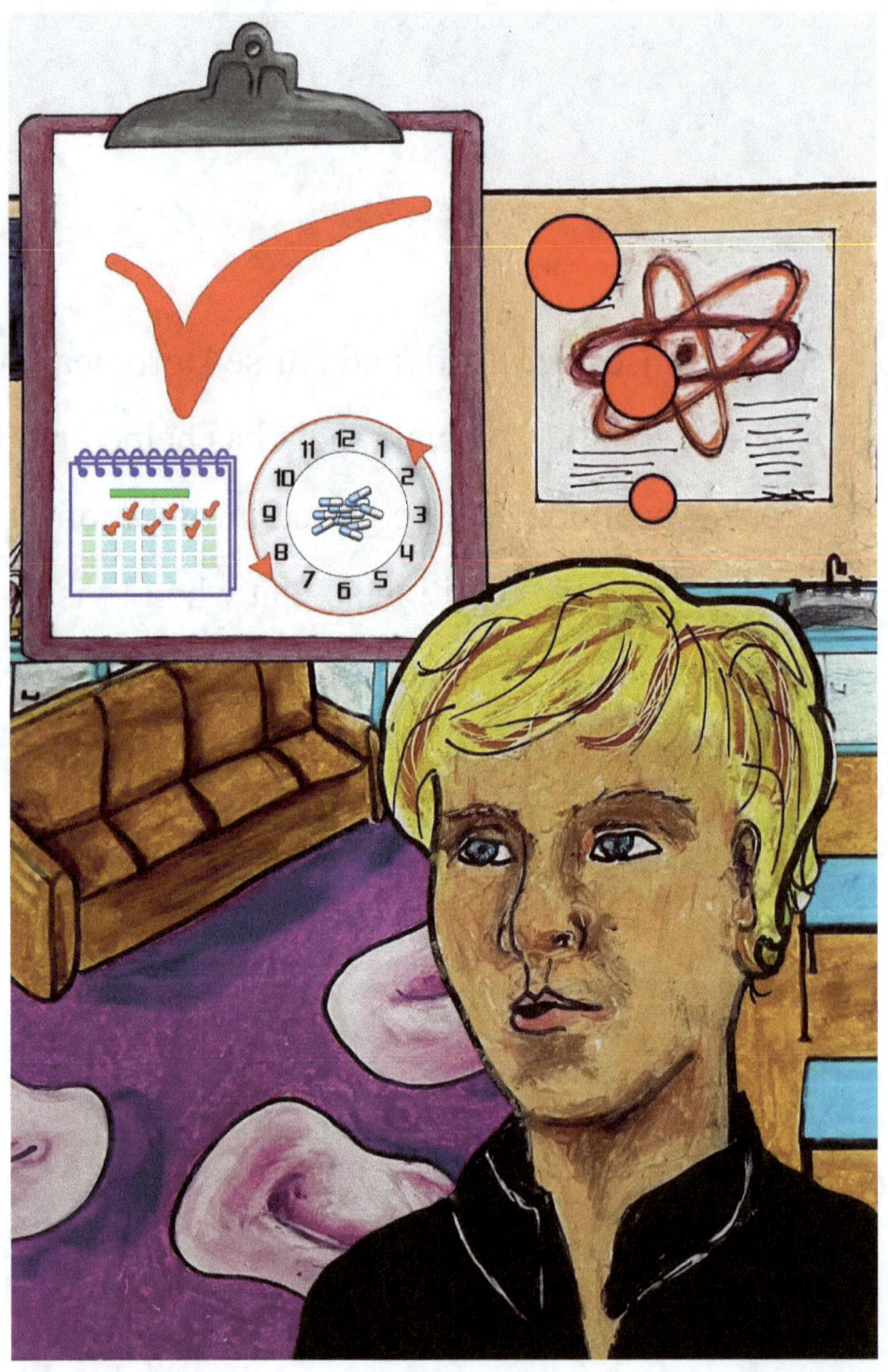

Dimitry raises his hand, and Nurse Dorothea calls on him to talk. "Social media has helped me stay compliant with my treatment. My Provider checks in with me using a special app, and that helps ensure I do what I'm supposed to do."

"Accountability is something we all have to learn, and having someone check up on you and make sure you stay accountable can be a good thing," says Nurse Dorothea.

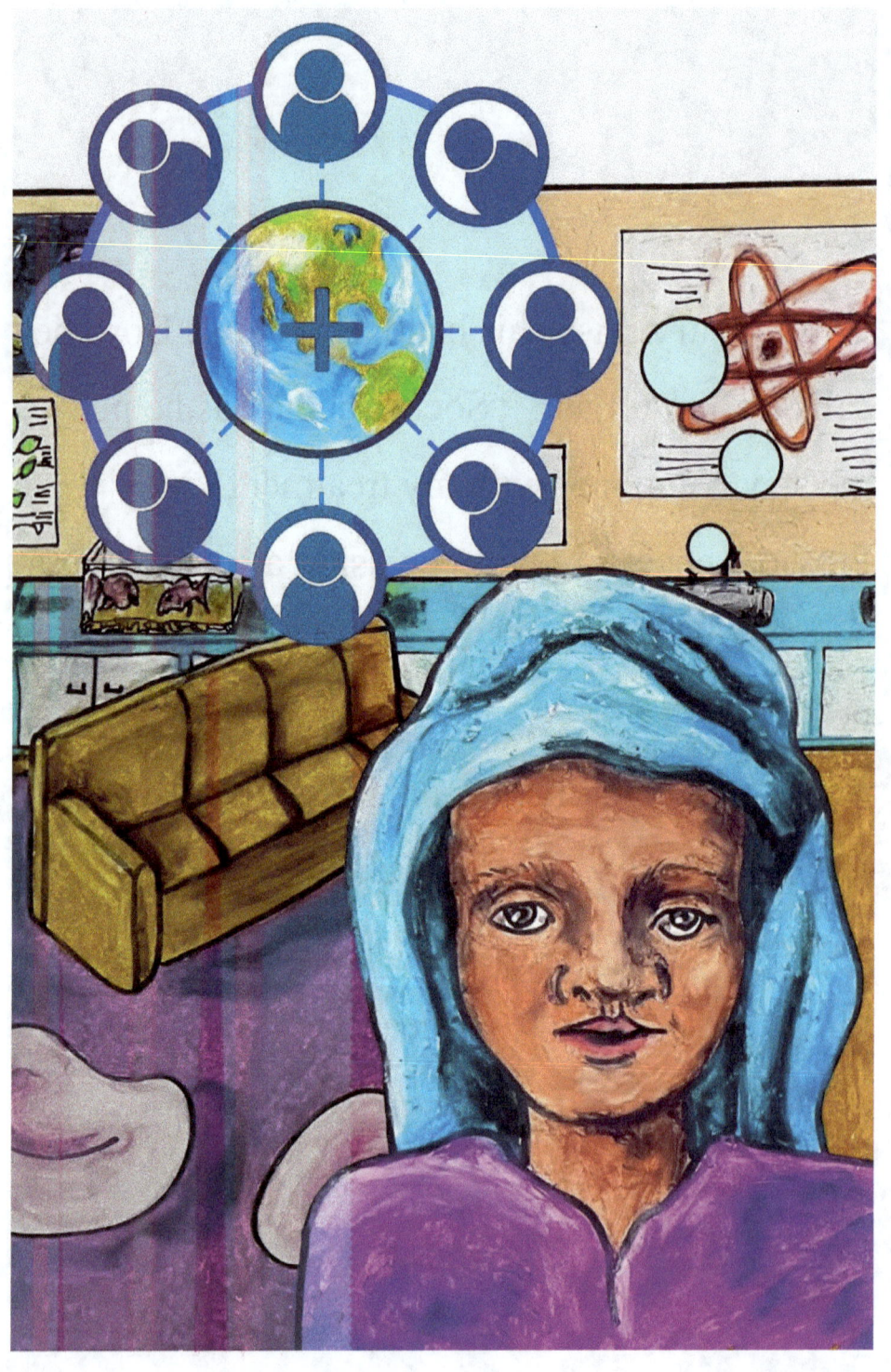

Yuliana raises her hand, and Nurse Dorothea calls on her to talk. "Social media has helped me feel more connected with the world. I have friends in several different countries, and I learn about their culture and the different things that impact their lives."

"The world is a big place, and we need to be accepting of each other's culture," says Nurse Dorothea.

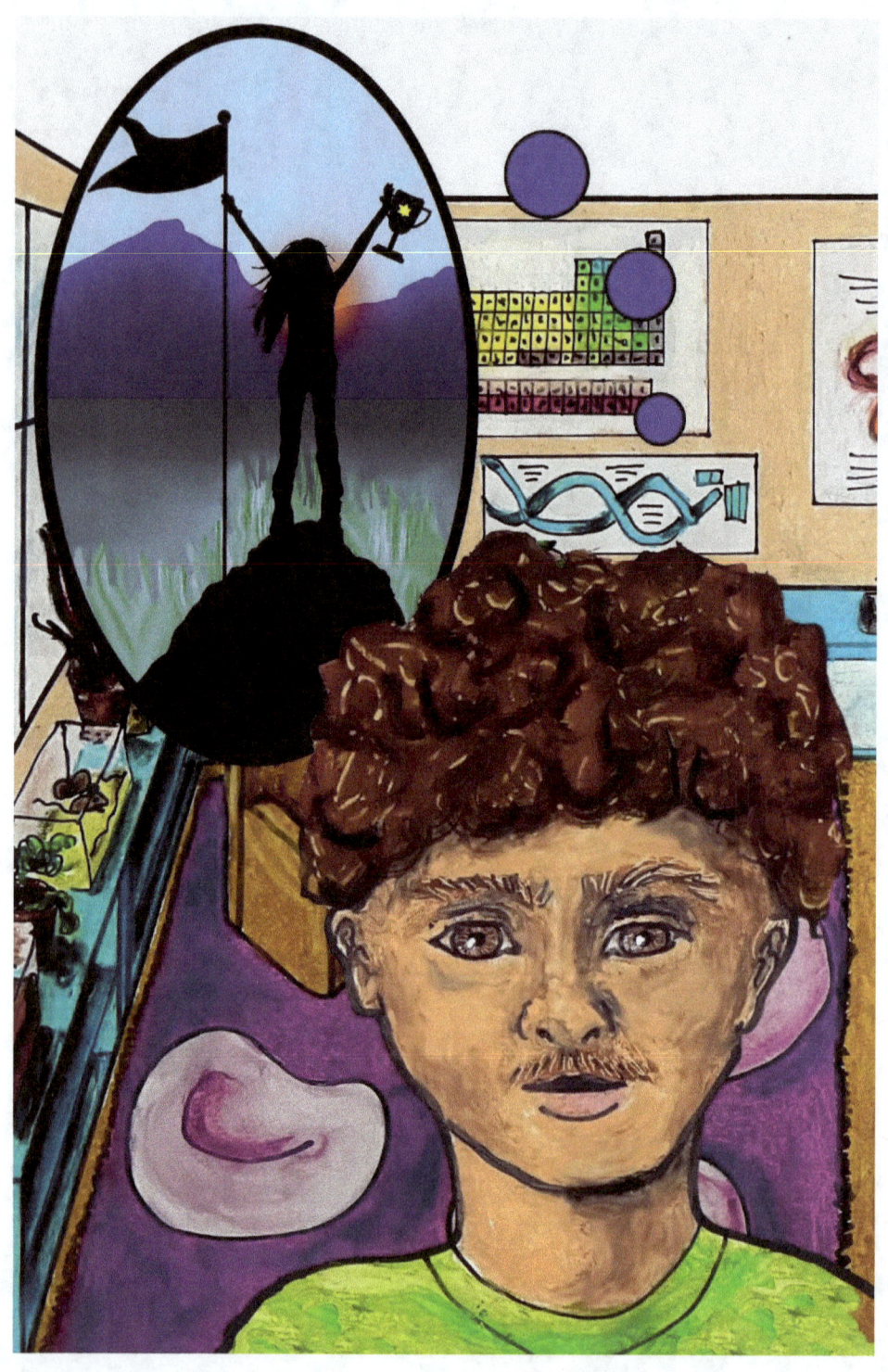

Gustavo raises his hand, and Nurse Dorothea calls on him to talk. "Social media helps me feel empowered and boosts my self-confidence so that I can do things and grow as a person."

"Seeing other examples of success online can help encourage us to become our best selves," says Nurse Dorothea.

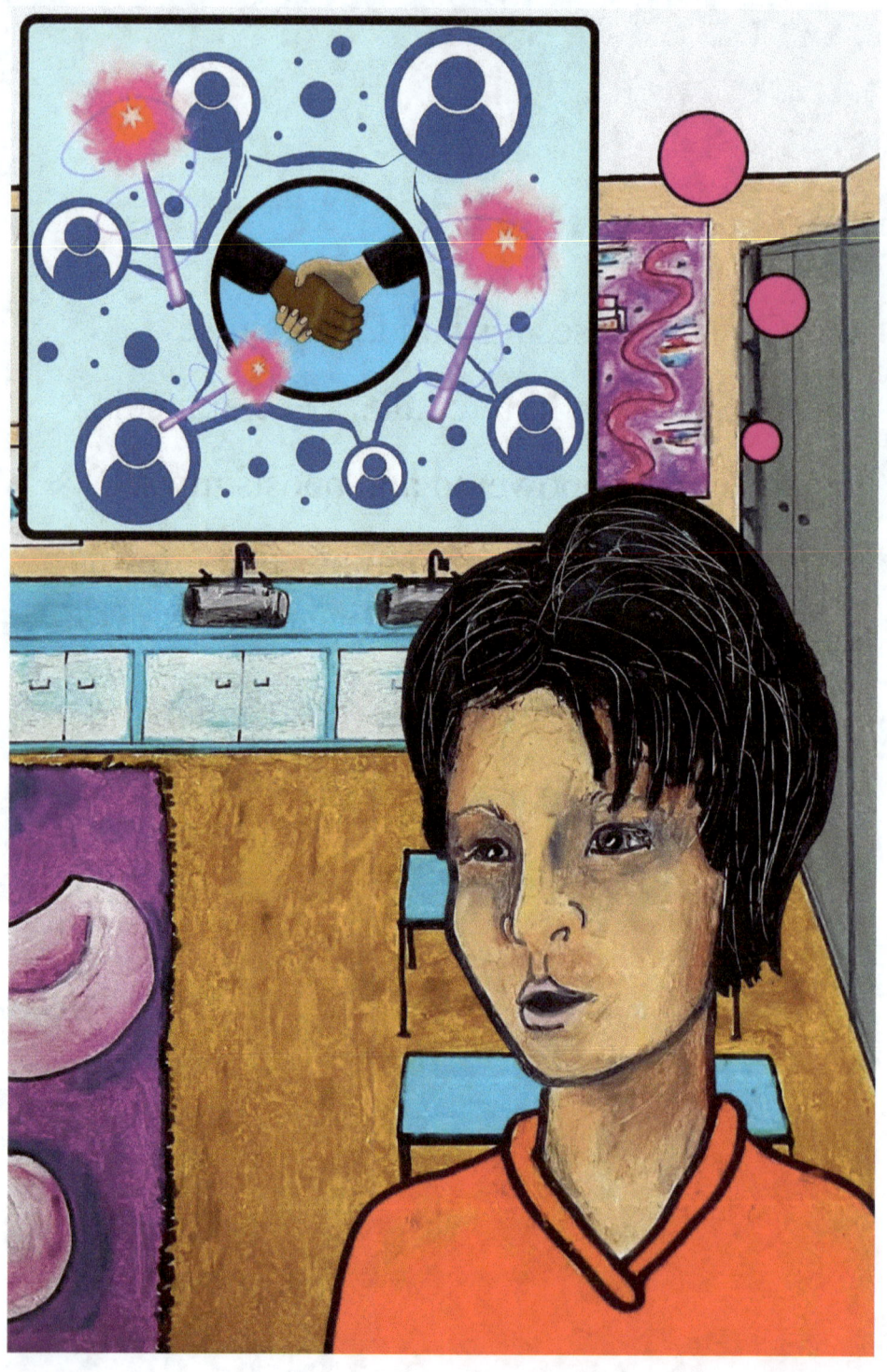

Kenji raises his hand, and Nurse Dorothea calls on him to talk. "I think social media has helped increase my social functioning. I think this will help me in my future career. I think it will help me become a better employee, co-worker, and mentor if I am put in that position."

"We are social creatures, so improving our interactions with others is a good thing and a necessity," says Nurse Dorothea.

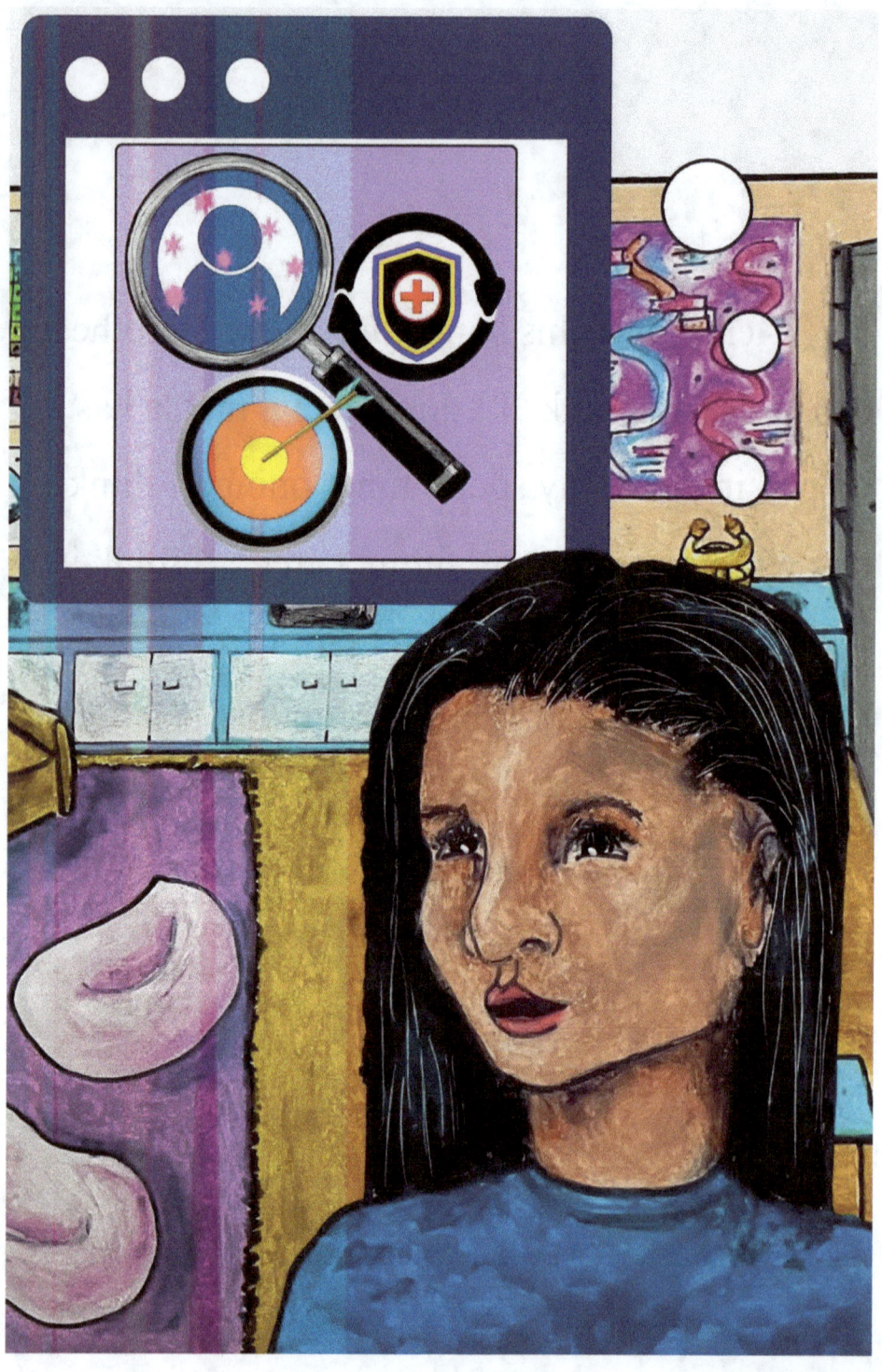

Diwa raises her hand, and Nurse Dorothea calls on her to talk. "I have an app that helps me monitor my symptoms, prevent relapses, and set goals. Managing my disease is a Godsend."

"Most of us will have a disease at some point in our lives so having something to help us to live a fuller life with a disease is very helpful," says Nurse Dorothea.

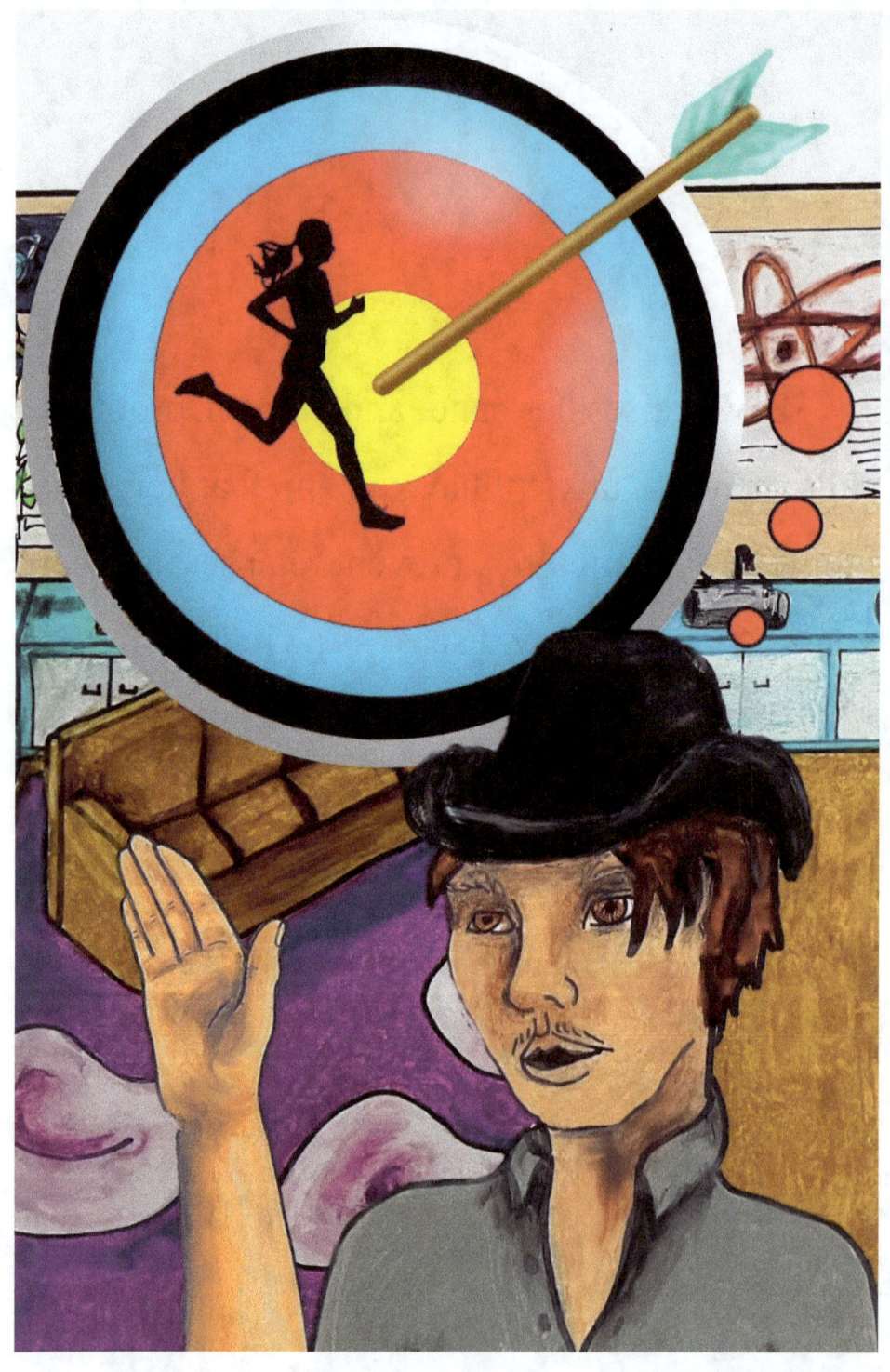

Wyatt raises his hand, and Nurse Dorothea calls on him to talk. "I use social media to accomplish my fitness goals. It helps me stay on target and do what I hope to do every week. My online community also helps me stay motivated to accomplish these goals."

"Regular exercise can help with mental health, so it is great that you are using social media to support your objectives," says Nurse Dorothea.

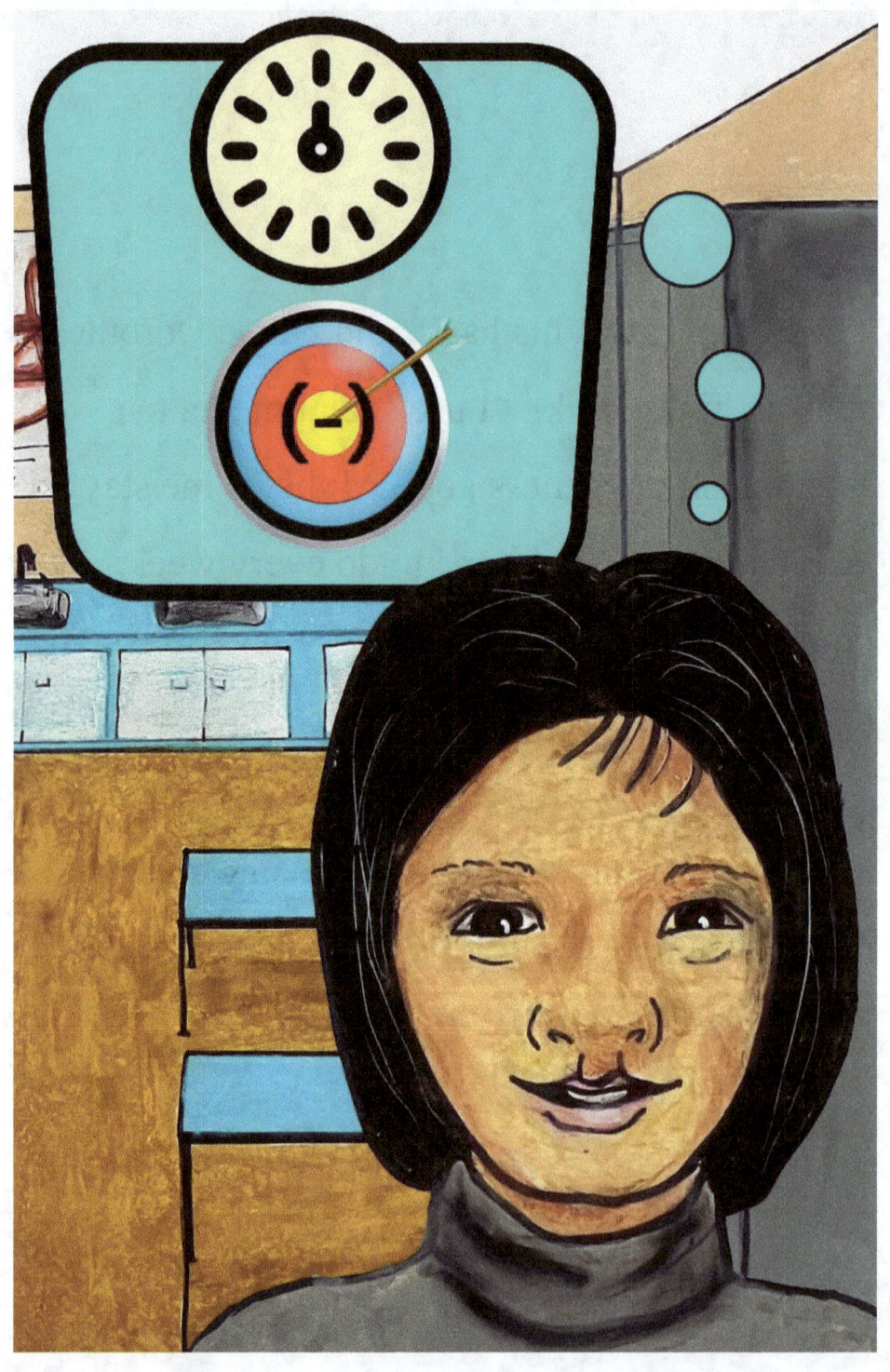

Lian raises her hand, and Nurse Dorothea calls on her to talk. "Social media has helped me accomplish my weight loss goals. I am now at a healthy weight, feel better about myself, feel less tired, and have more hope for the future."

"Living a healthy life is important for your mental health," says Nurse Dorothea.

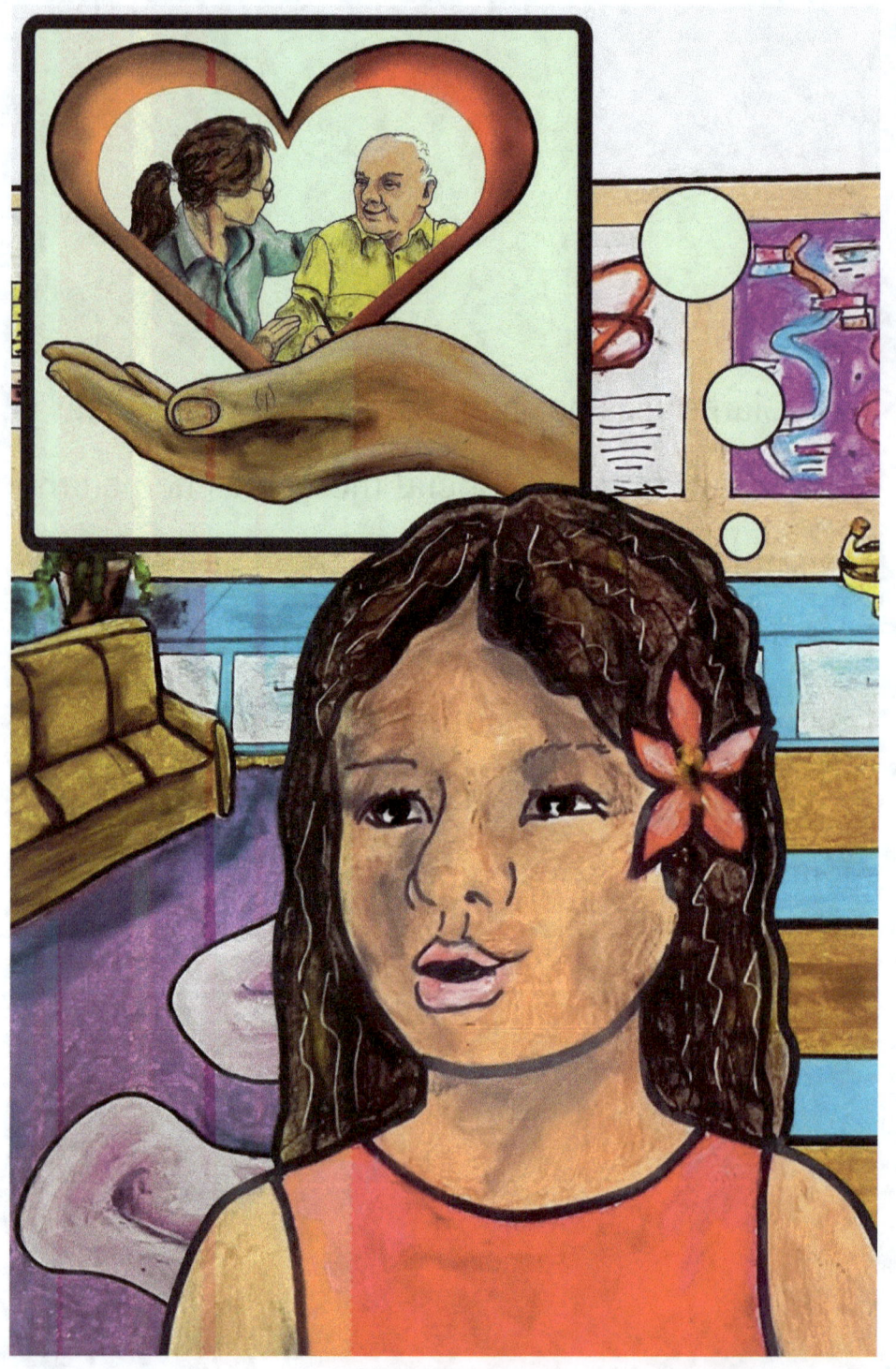

Kalani raises her hand, and Nurse Dorothea calls on her to talk. "I have seen family members get the online support they need when they are helping others. My mom gets a lot of encouragement and support as she helps my granddad with dementia."

"Caregiver support is important and necessary to help families live a higher quality life," says Nurse Dorothea.

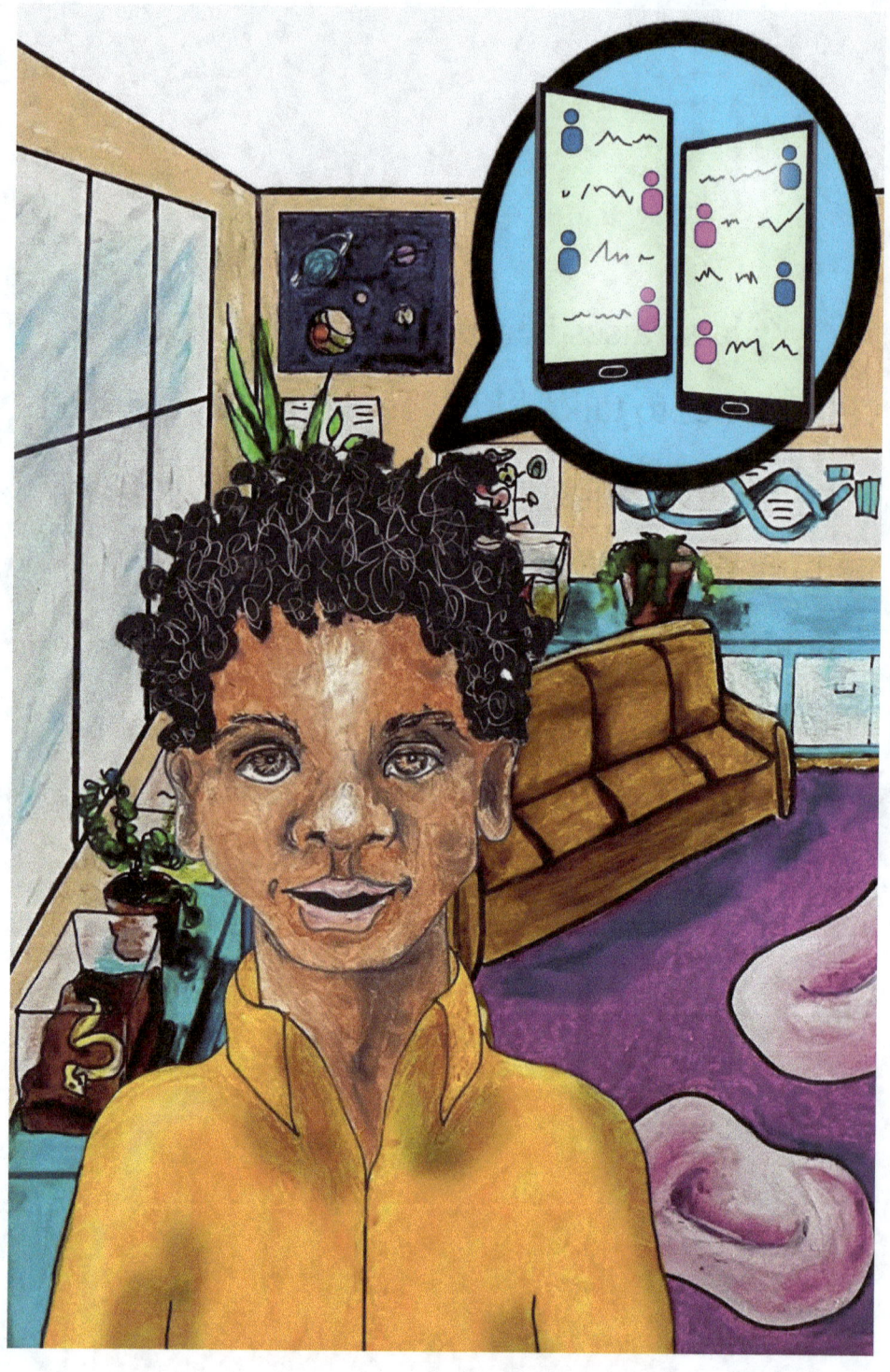

Amari raises his hand, and Nurse Dorothea calls on him to talk. "I think instant communication is really neat. It helps me stay connected to my friends in real-time so that I know what is going on with everyone."

"Instant communication is really helpful when there is breaking news that many people need to know about. It is also a great way to stay connected to family and friends that live far away," says Nurse Dorothea.

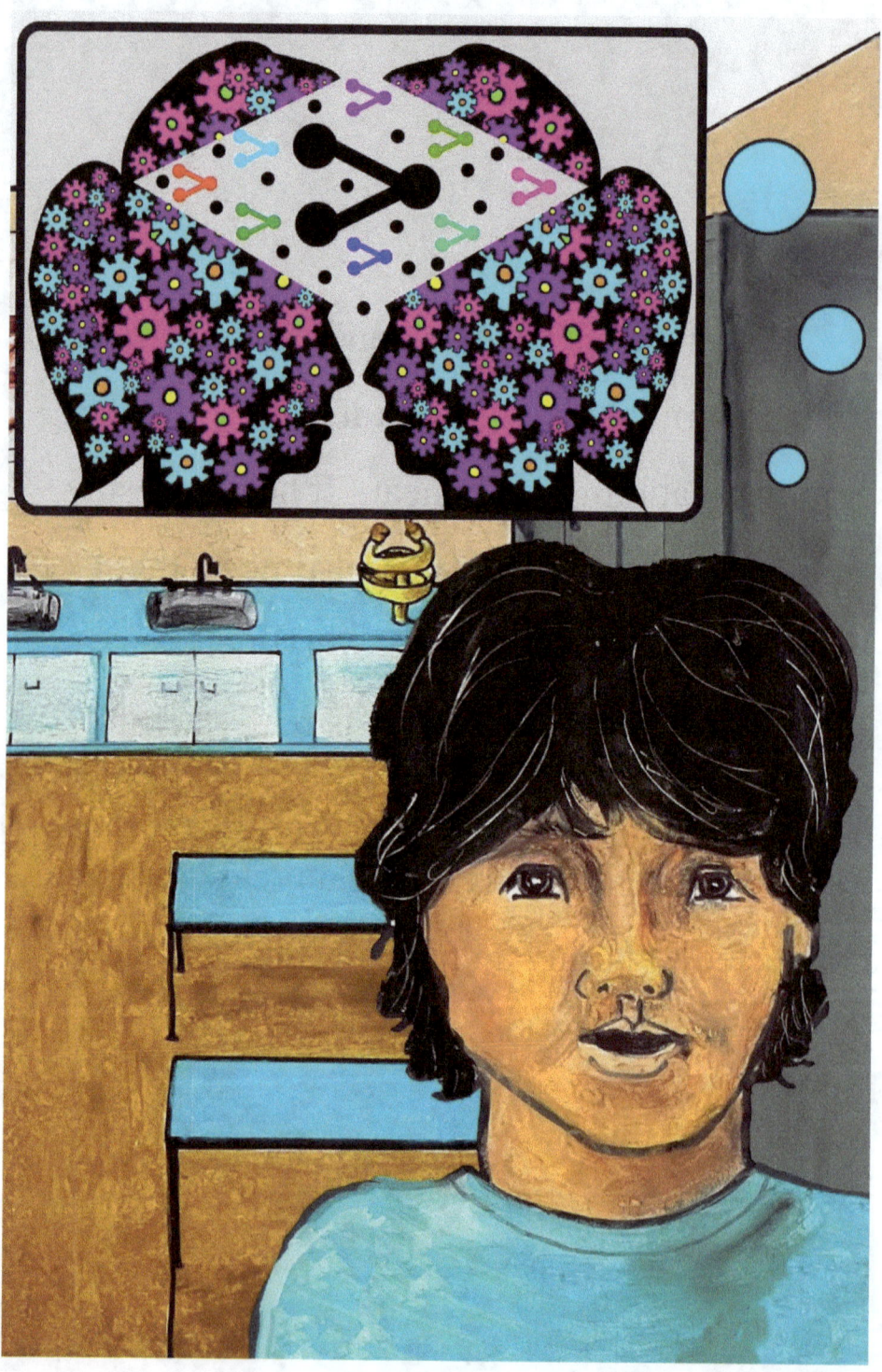

Ji Ho raises his hand, and Nurse Dorothea calls on him to talk. "Knowledge sharing is a great thing about social media. Sharing knowledge with others helps people make more informed and better decisions for their lives."

"Yes, getting more info so that you make a better decision can help avoid failure and ensure success in your future," says Nurse Dorothea.

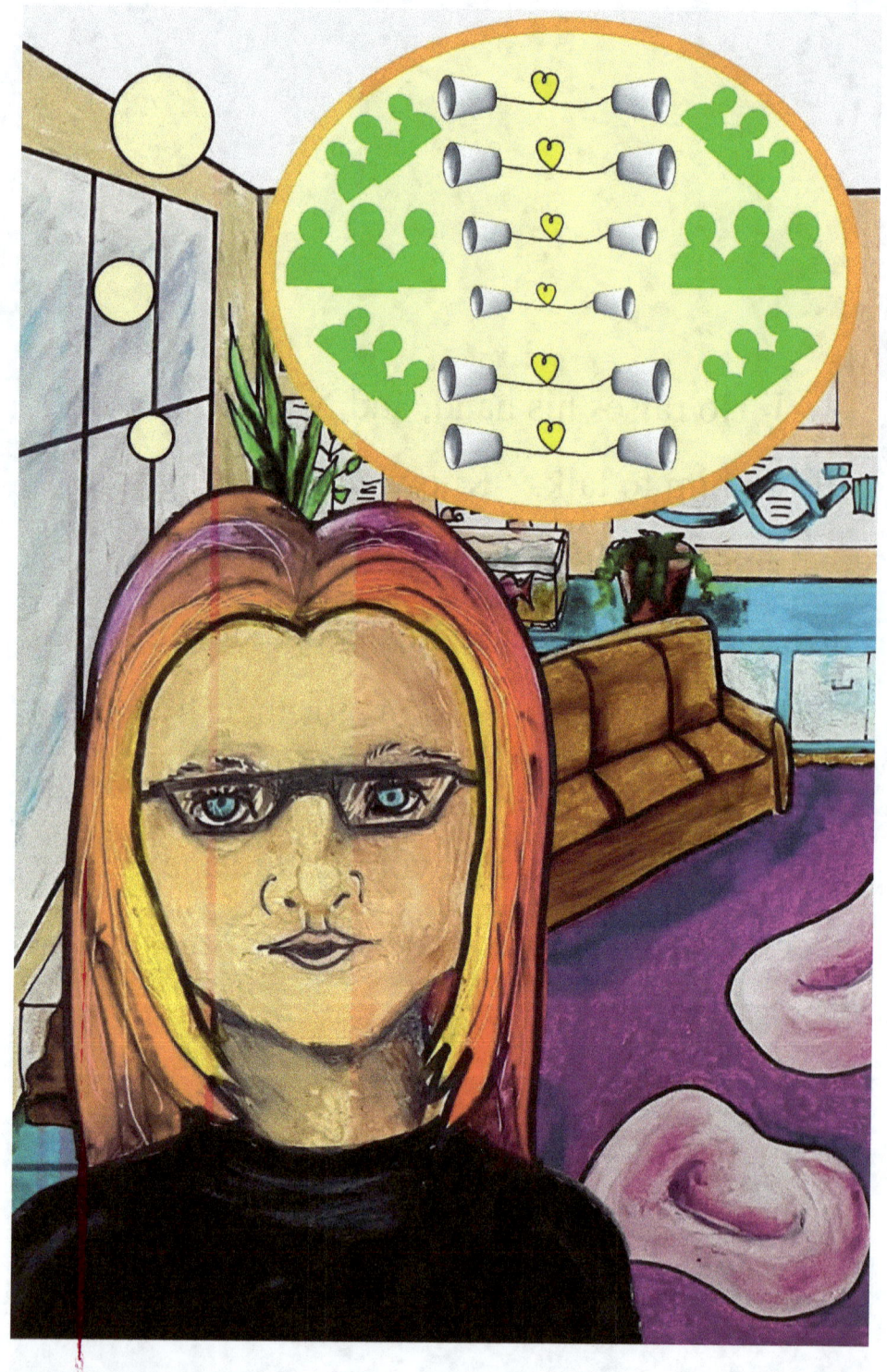

Juniper raises her hand, and Nurse Dorothea calls on her to talk. "Social media has helped me stay in touch with old friends."

"Let me tell you, having some old friends that have known you most of your life is an important thing. It helps create a sense of personal integrity and helps give feedback on how you are doing as a person since these old friends know all your ups and downs. I know you may not stay in touch with all your friends once you graduate high school, but try hard to stay in touch with some," says Nurse Dorothea.

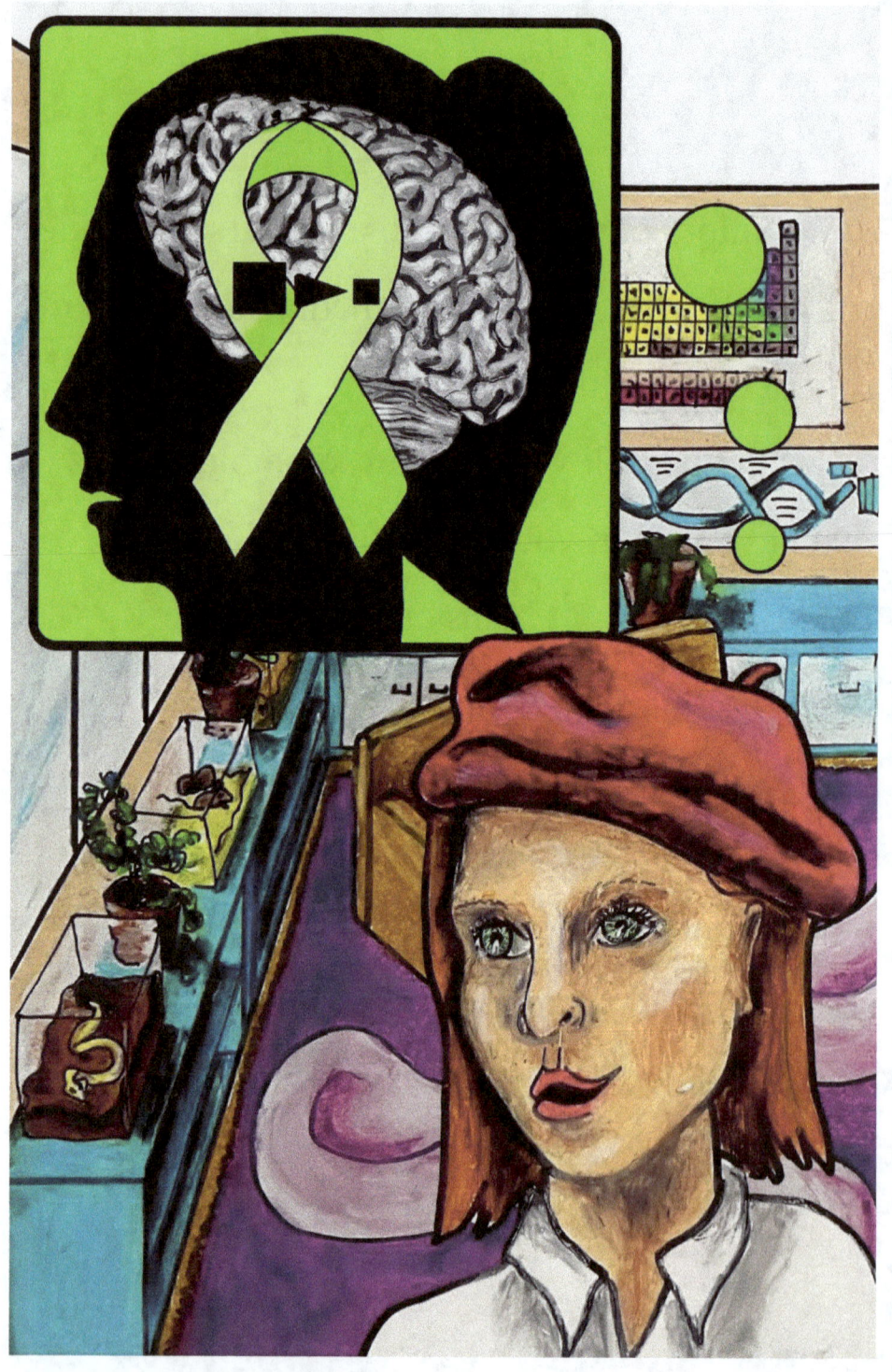

Maria raises her hand, and Nurse Dorothea calls on her to talk. "I think social media reduces stigma against certain groups of people."

"You're correct. When we talk about certain conditions without judgment and learn about each other in a safe space, we can come together and be more accepting in our non-digital world," says Nurse Dorothea.

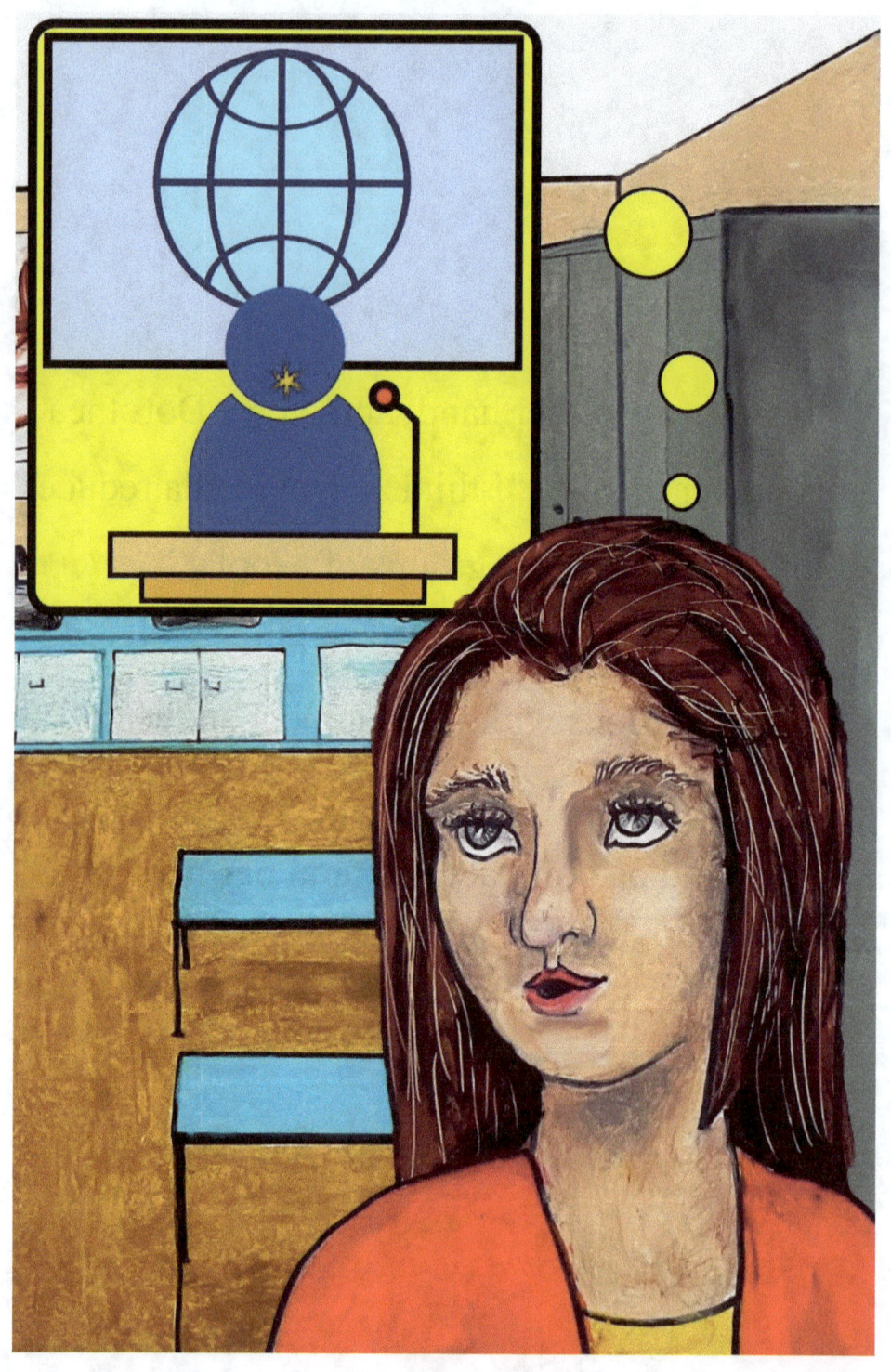

Awira raises her hand, and Nurse Dorothea calls on her to talk. "Social media can help us prepare for disasters by sharing news about upcoming events like potential hurricanes in certain areas. The more we know, the more we can prepare for bad things."

"Excellent point. Social media can be used to warn us of dangers," says Nurse Dorothea.

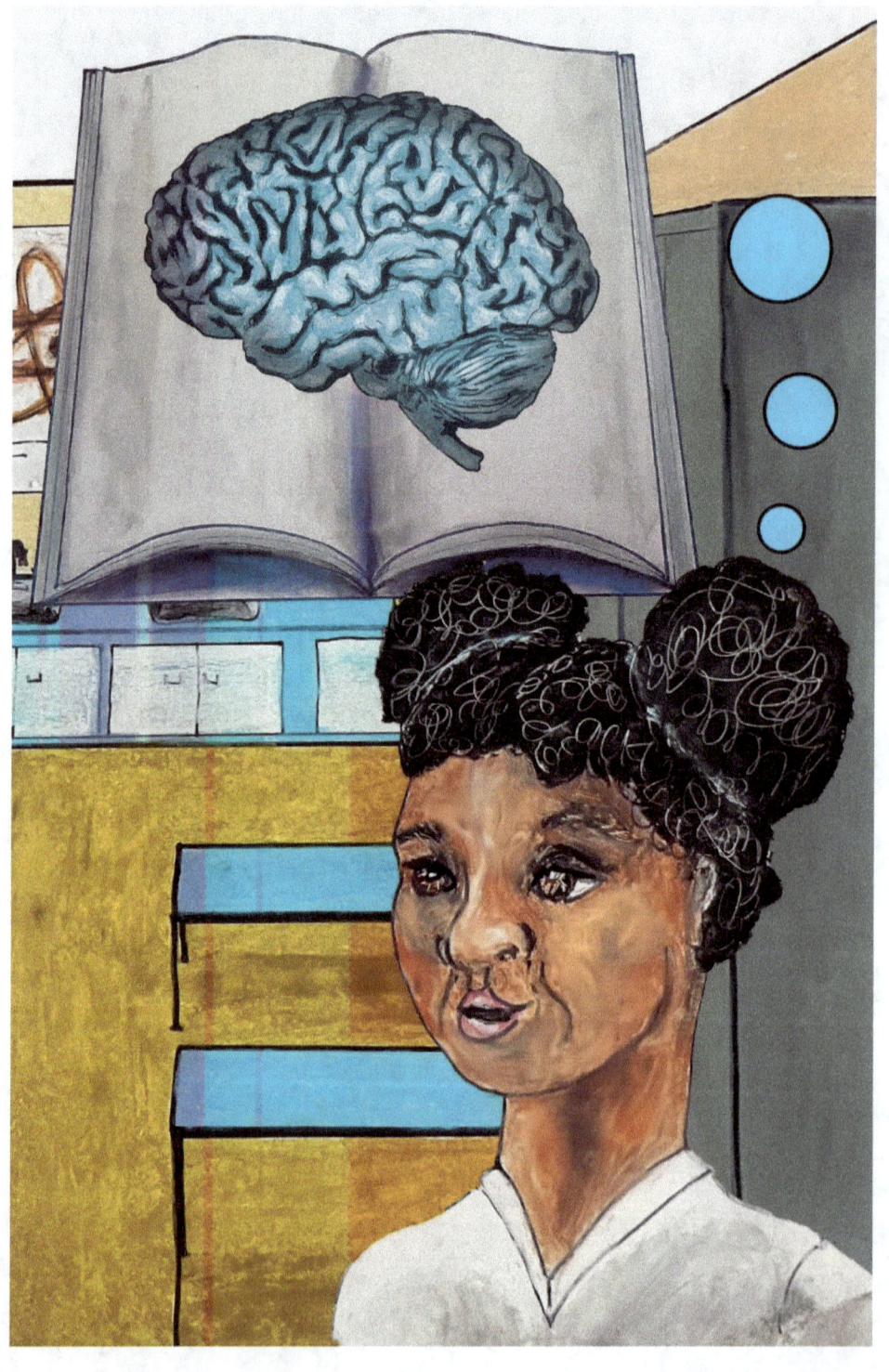

Amisha raises her hand, and Nurse Dorothea calls on her to talk. "Social media promotes learning. The more ideas we have, the more options we can have in our lives to do the best things for ourselves and our community."

"Science has helped advance our knowledge in big ways, and sharing advances of science with others through social media can help us achieve our full potential," says Nurse Dorothea.

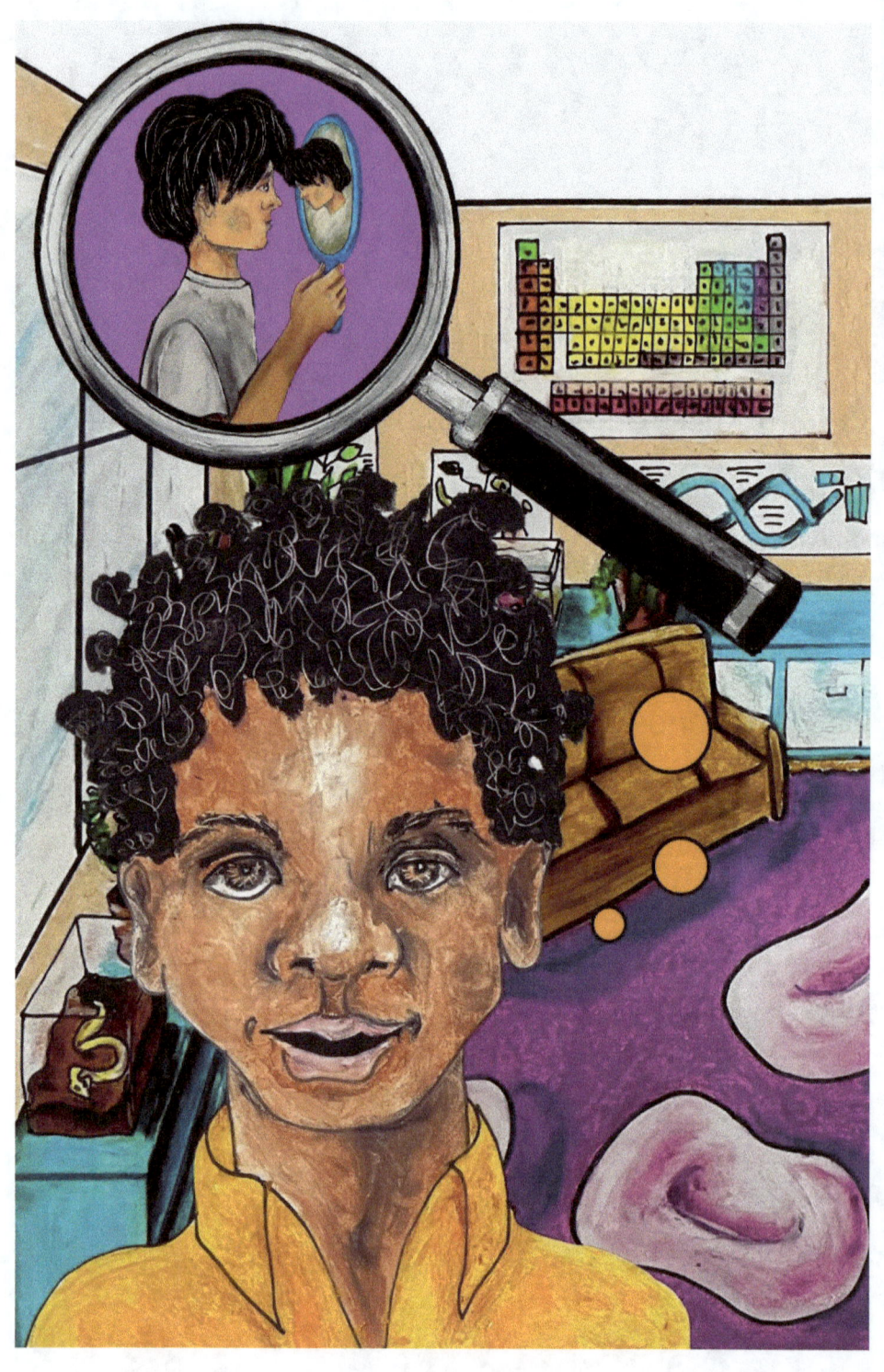

Amari raises his hand, and Nurse Dorothea calls on him to talk. "I think social media has helped me to find myself. I'm on a journey and am always learning."

"Life is a journey, and one of the nicest things is that we have someone in our life who is complex which is ourselves, and it can be fun to be alone and get to know oneself," says Nurse Dorothea.

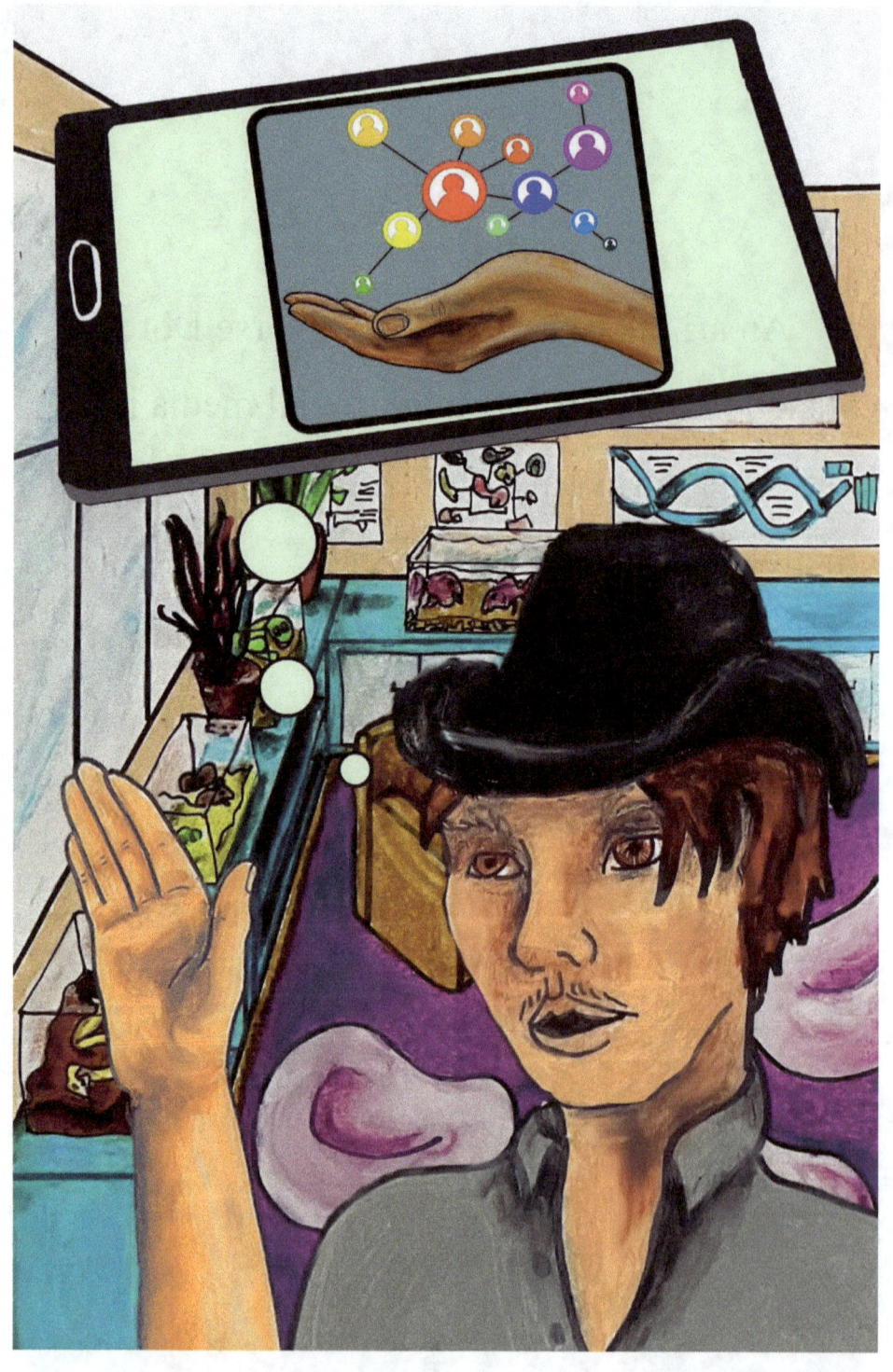

Wyatt raises his hand, and Nurse Dorothea calls on him to talk. "Social media increases access to social support. I love having a lot of people in my life who all help me out in different ways."

"It takes a community to grow up and thrive. It's important to flourish in life, not just survive," says Nurse Dorothea.

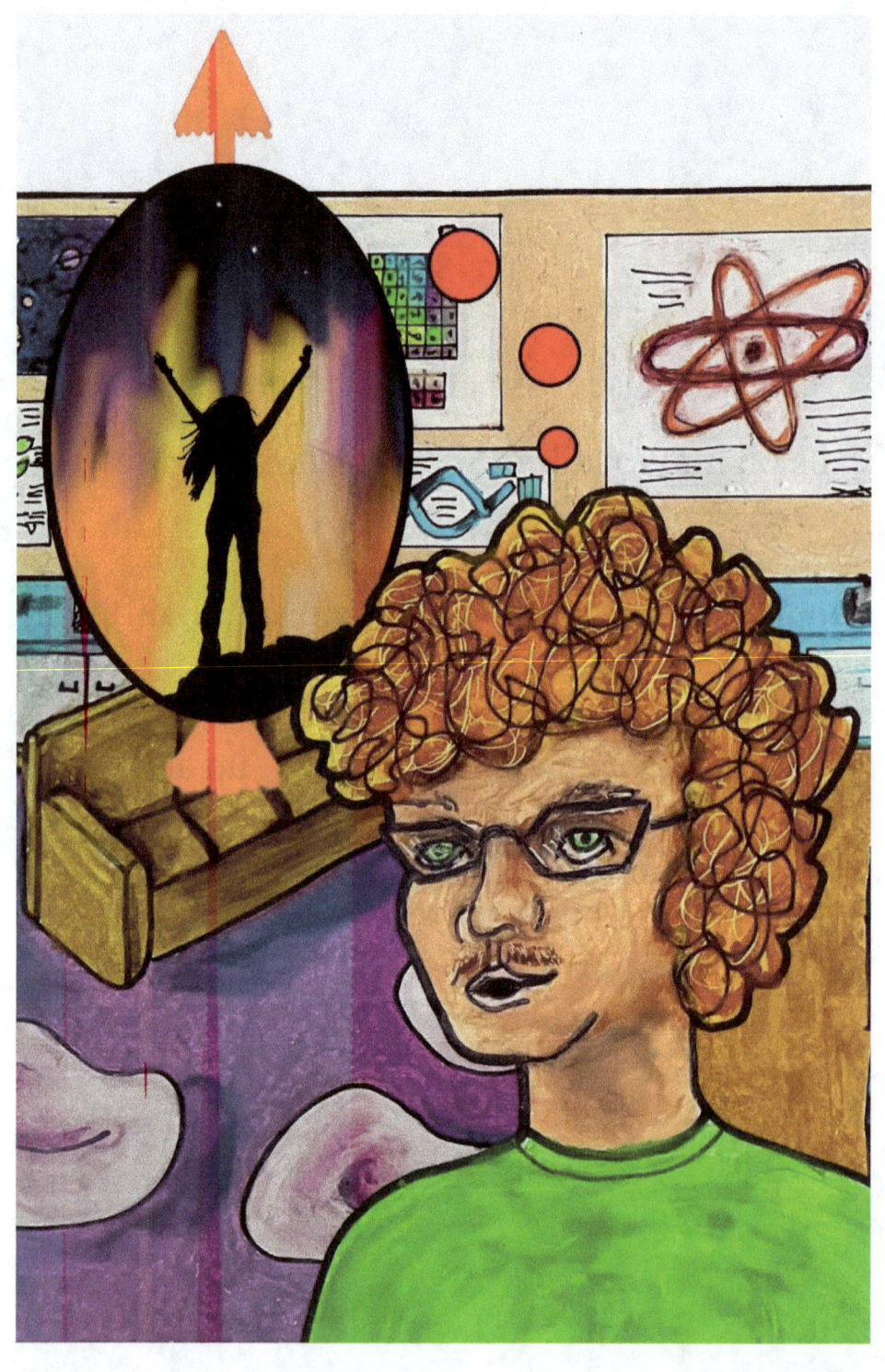

Connor raises his hand, and Nurse Dorothea calls on him to talk. "I think social media and interacting with others has boosted my happiness."

"That is good to hear," says Nurse Dorothea.

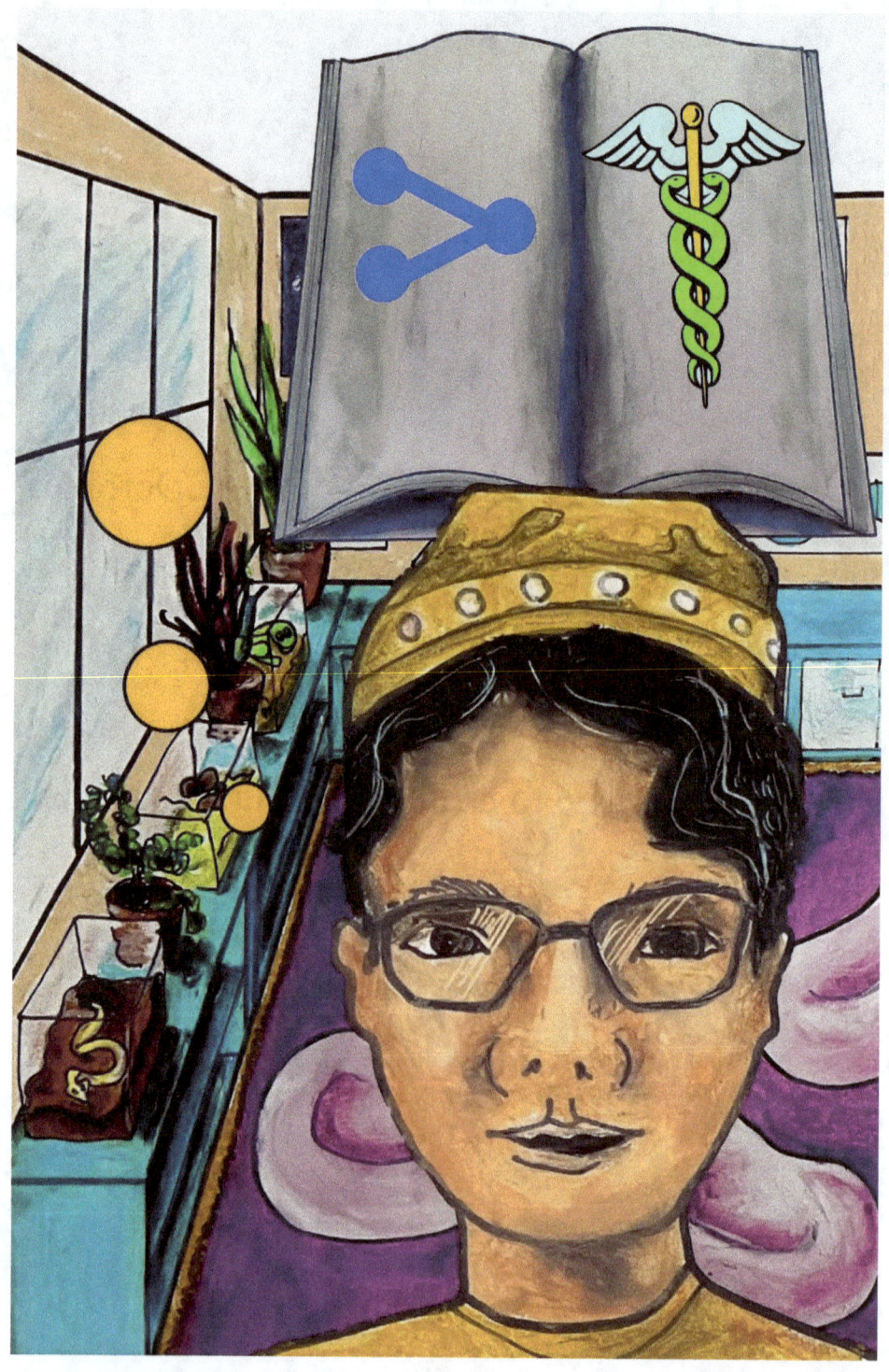

Azamat raises his hand, and Nurse Dorothea calls on him to talk. "I've used social media to learn about health and how to live a healthier life."

"Trust me, there seems to always be something we are learning about the body and how best to live a healthy life. Staying a lifelong learner is very important," says Nurse Dorothea.

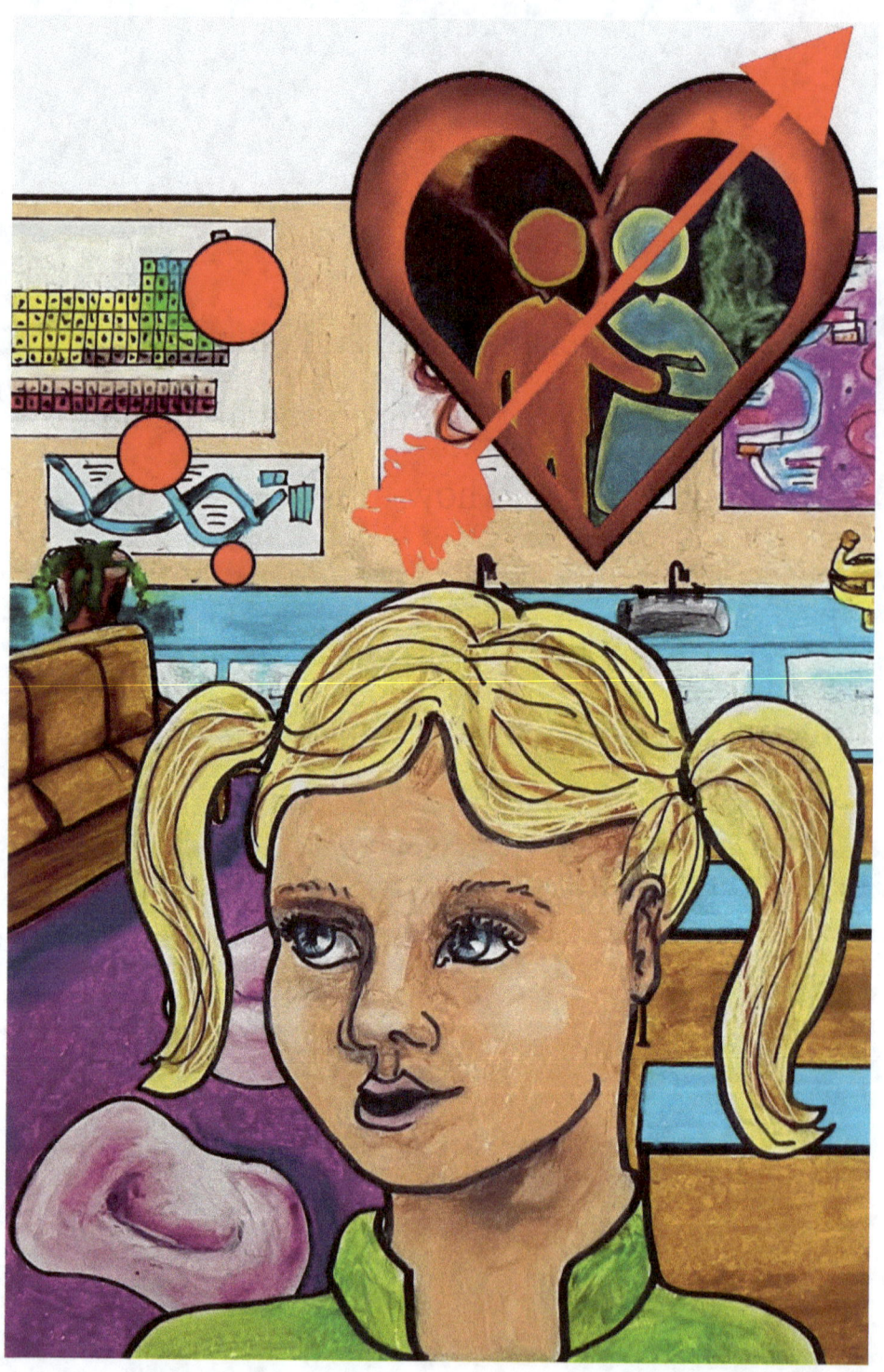

Frida raises her hand, and Nurse Dorothea calls on her to talk. "Social media has helped promote a loving relationship with my partner. It has helped us to stay connected and to give us ideas on what else we can do to have a stronger relationship"

"Relationships take a lot of effort to maintain," says Nurse Dorothea.

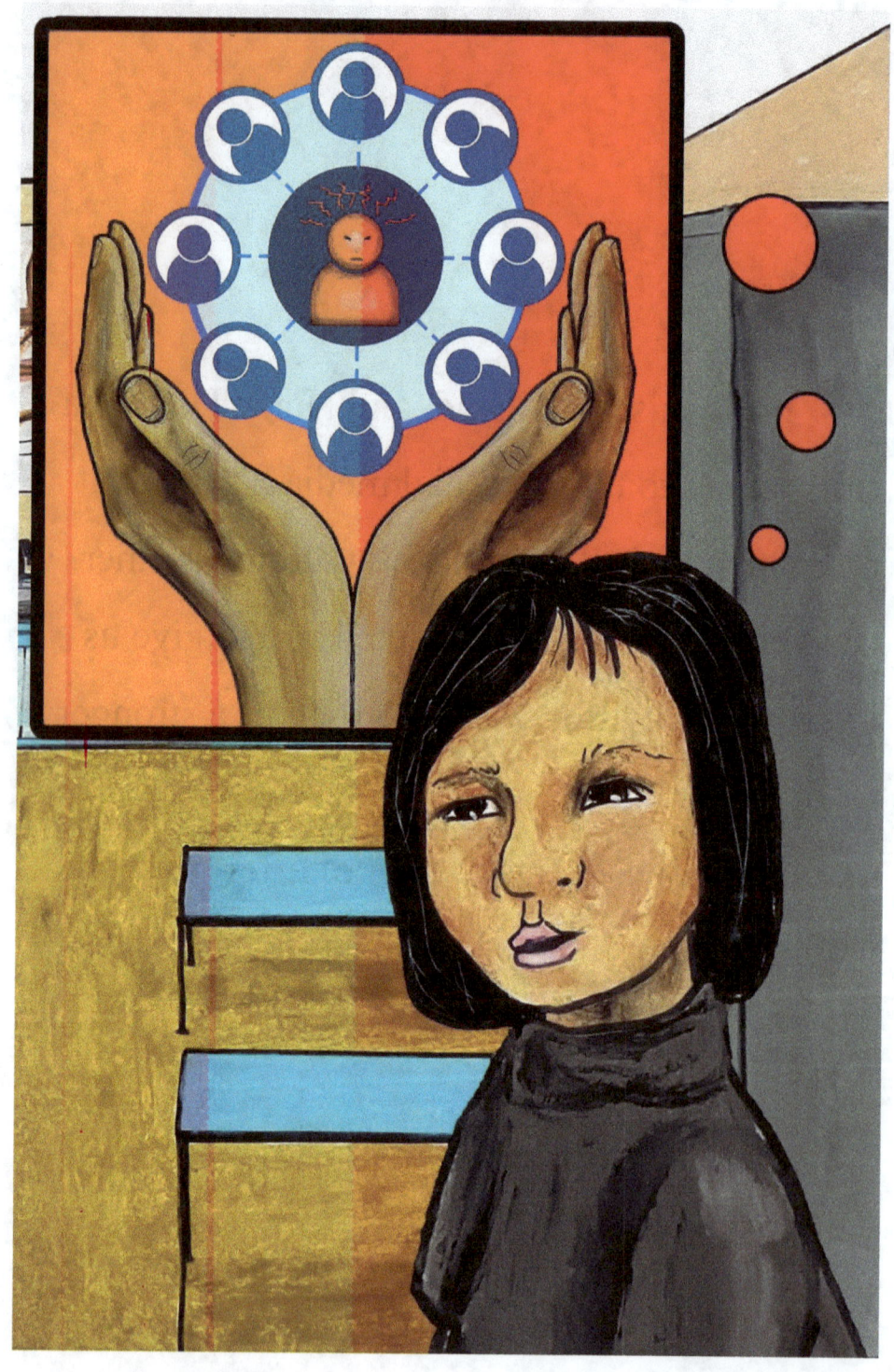

Lian raises her hand, and Nurse Dorothea calls on her to talk. "Social media supports me when I'm stressed. I connect with people that offer nice words to comfort me, and I also get presented ideas to solutions to my problems so that I can effectively deal with the issues in my life."

"Stress relief is important since too much stress can often trigger some diseases," says Nurse Dorothea.

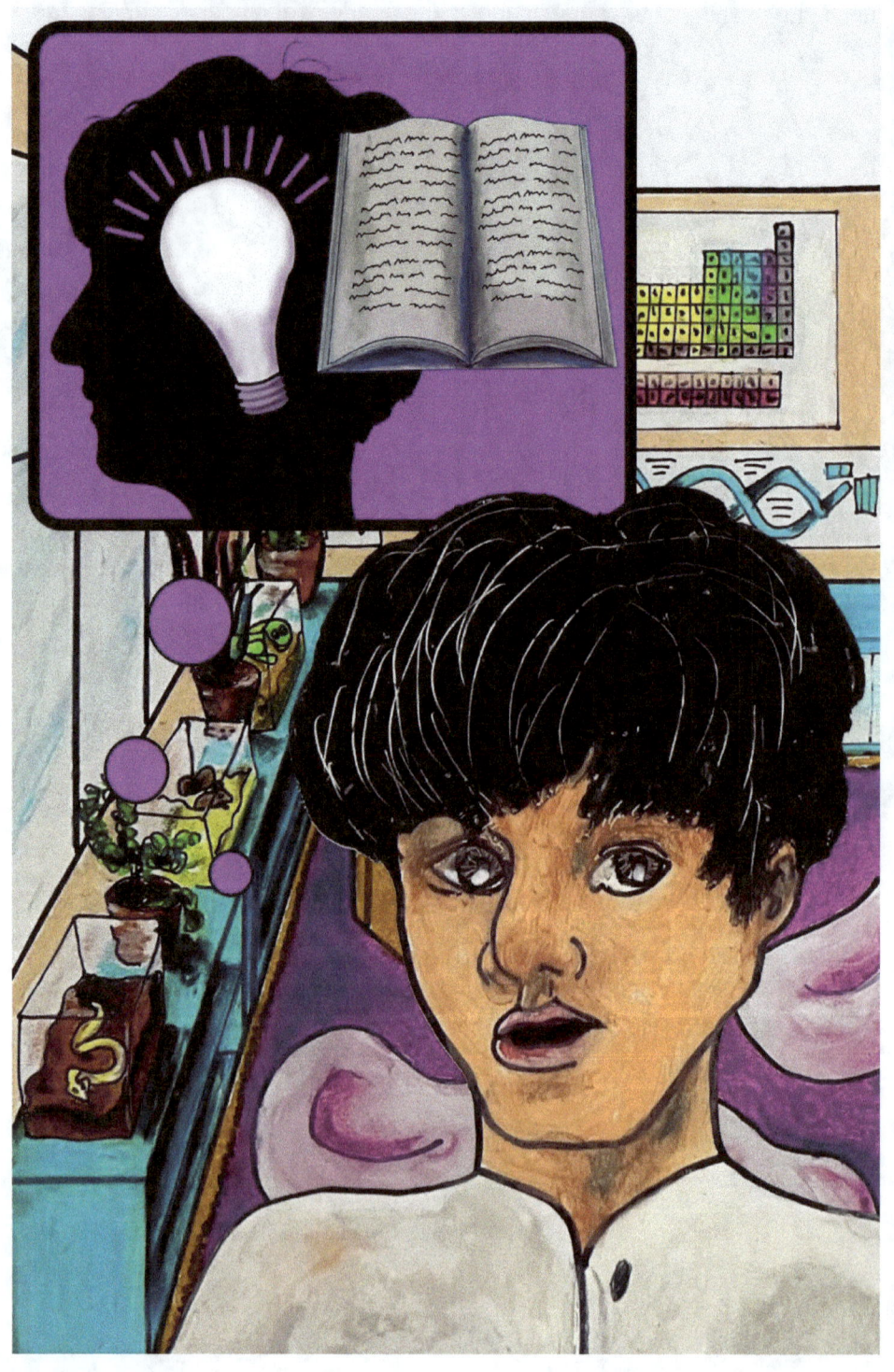

Antonio raises his hand, and Nurse Dorothea calls on him to talk. "Social media has helped me be an active learner. I see things that spark my interest and then do research on my own to discover new worlds of ideas. I interact with the information so that I learn even more than just passively reading something."

"That is really neat," says Nurse Dorothea.

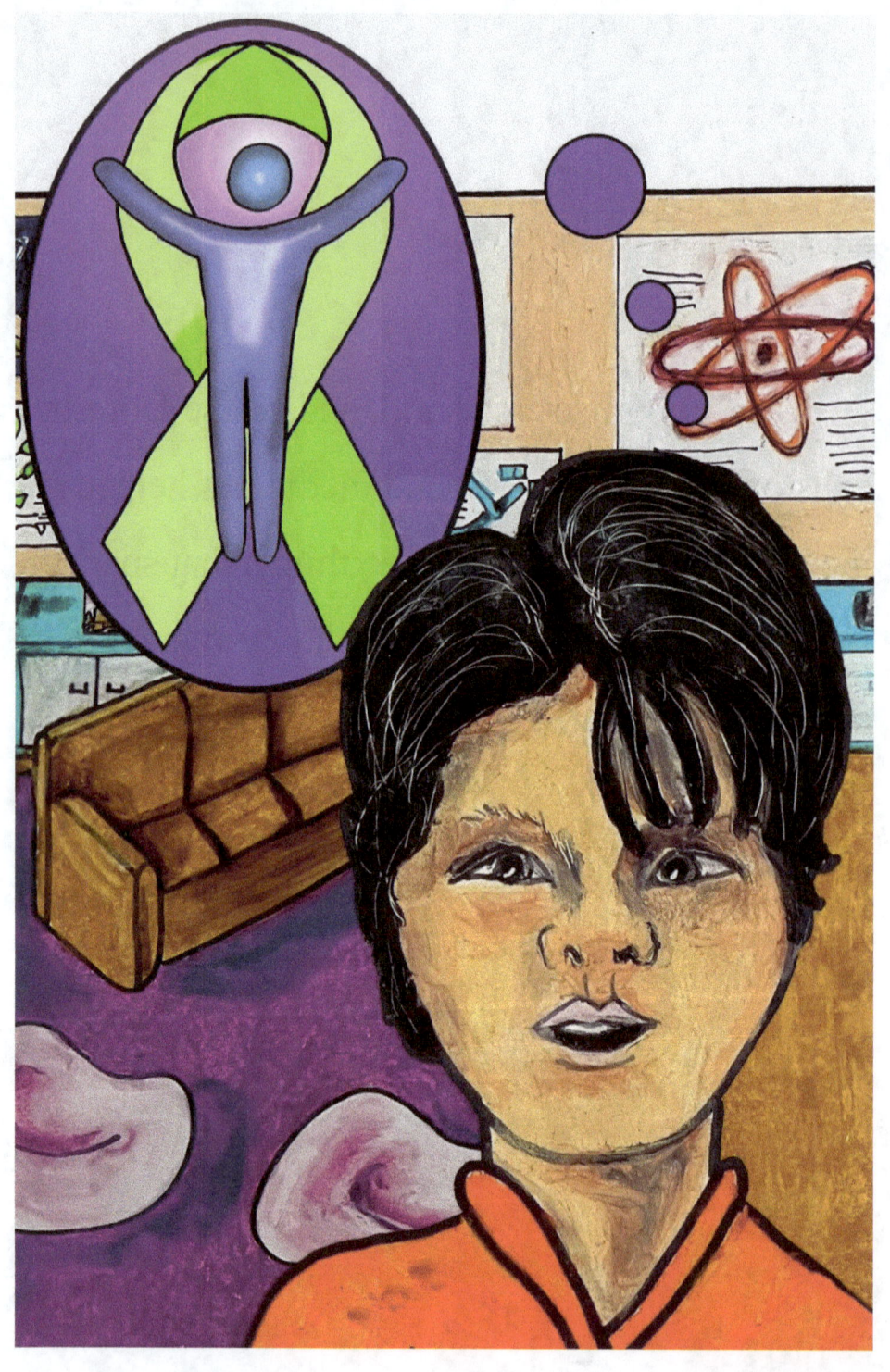

Kenji raises his hand, and Nurse Dorothea calls on him to talk. "I've used social media to promote not just my well-being, but also the well-being of my family and friends. I like to share tips each month that have helped me."

"We never know how many people we could touch with our words. You could be promoting well-being to many others you may never meet in person," says Nurse Dorothea.

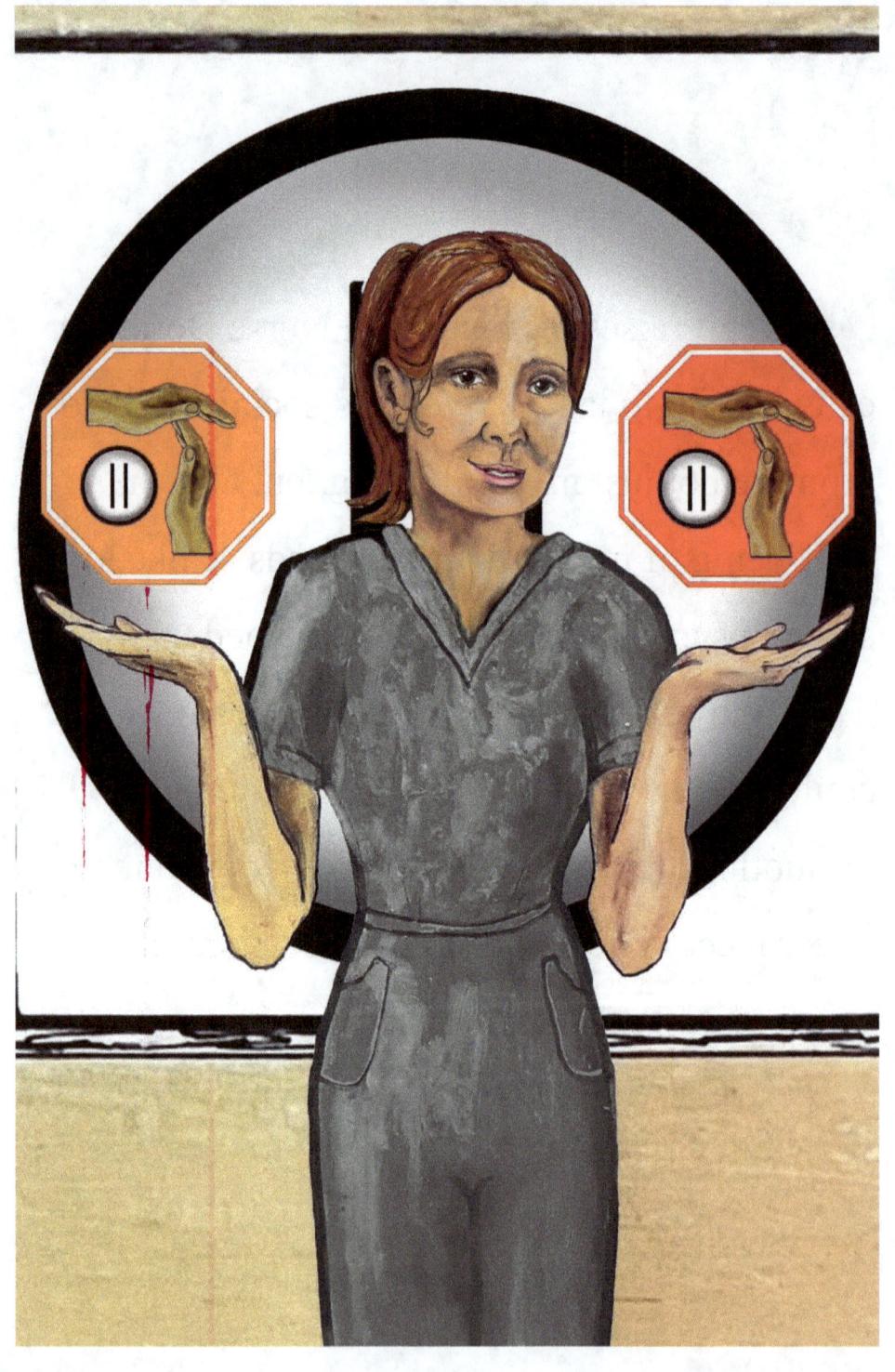

"We have gone over a lot of material. I would like you to refresh yourselves. We'll start again shortly after our break. For those watching the show or reading the book, feel free to stop here and start the next part when you are ready."

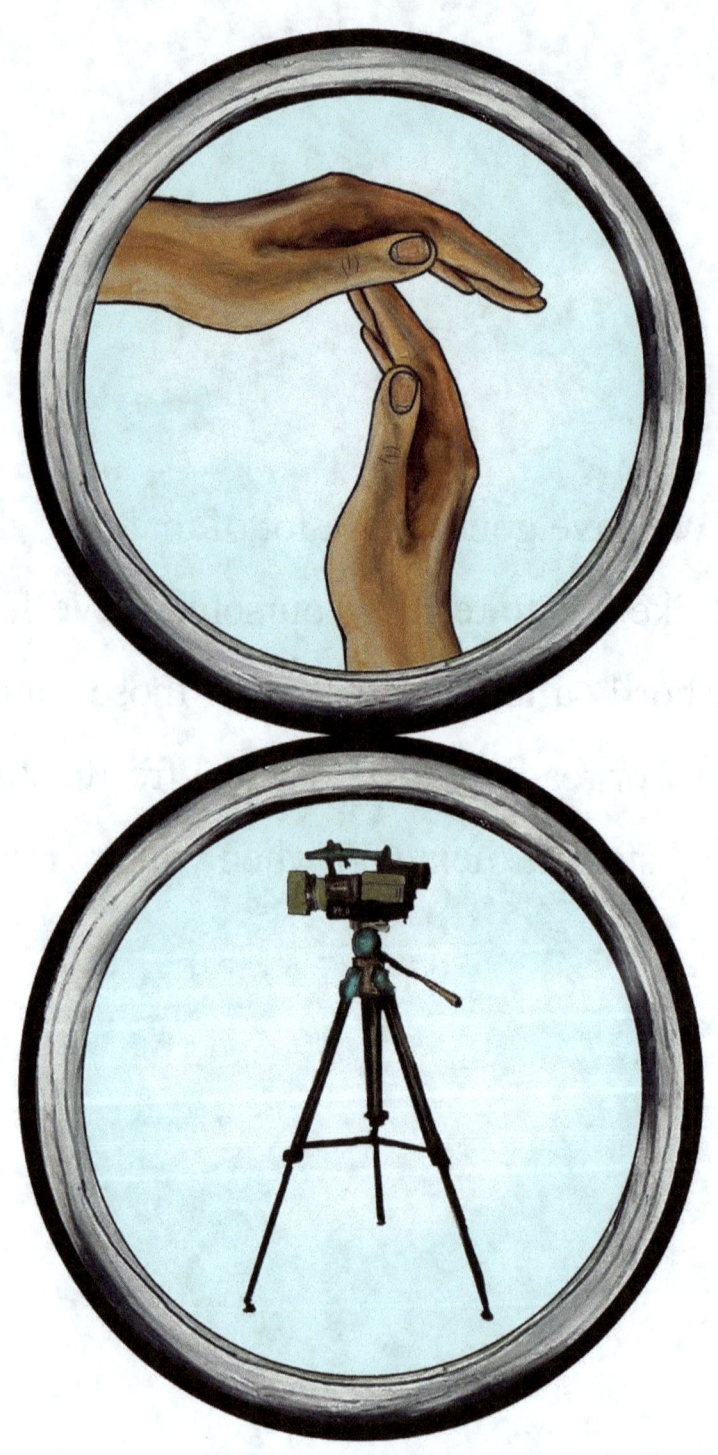

Part 2

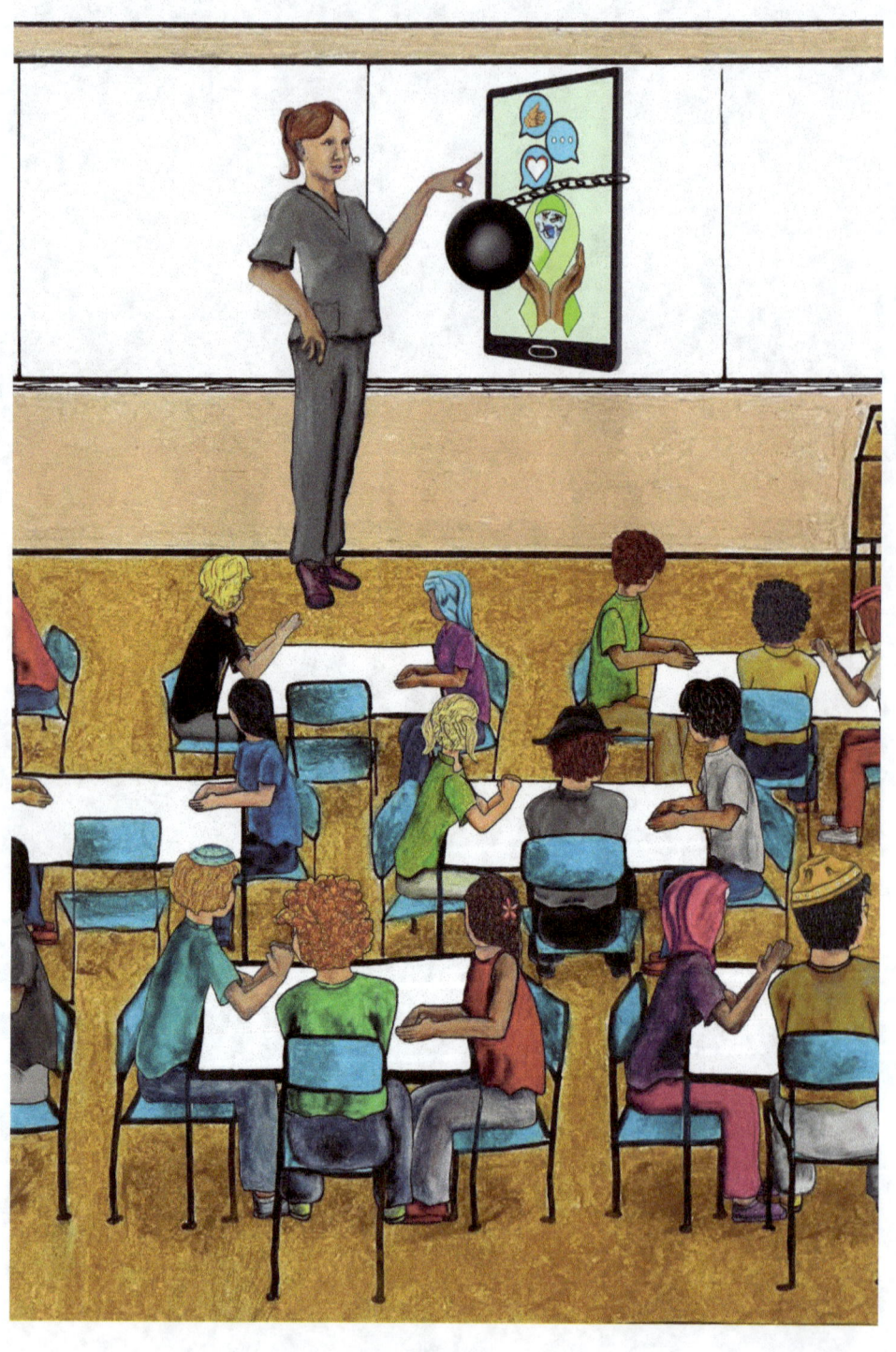

"Welcome back. Now, let's talk about symptoms that may show you are addicted to social media. One symptom is having a craving and feeling like you cannot go without it. If a person has emotional discomfort when they cut back on the time they use social media, then they may be addicted. Another symptom is being unable to cut back on the time you spend. If you have conflicts in your relationships due to the time you spend on social media, then you may be addicted," says Nurse Dorothea.

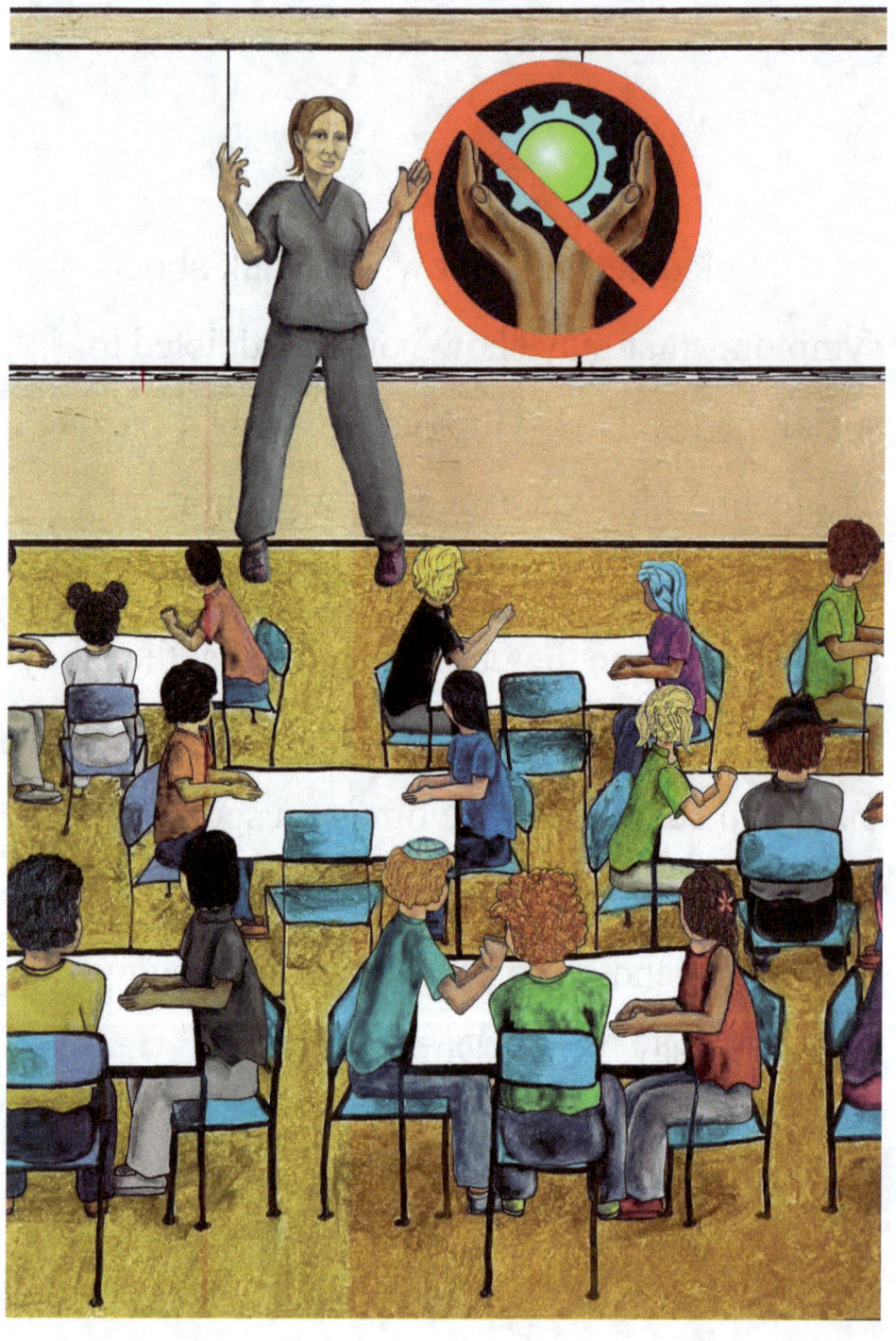

"If your social media usage impairs your ability to do other things, then you should be concerned. If you continue to use social media even though you realize it is damaging relationships and preventing you from accomplishing necessary goals in your life, then you may be addicted," says Nurse Dorothea.

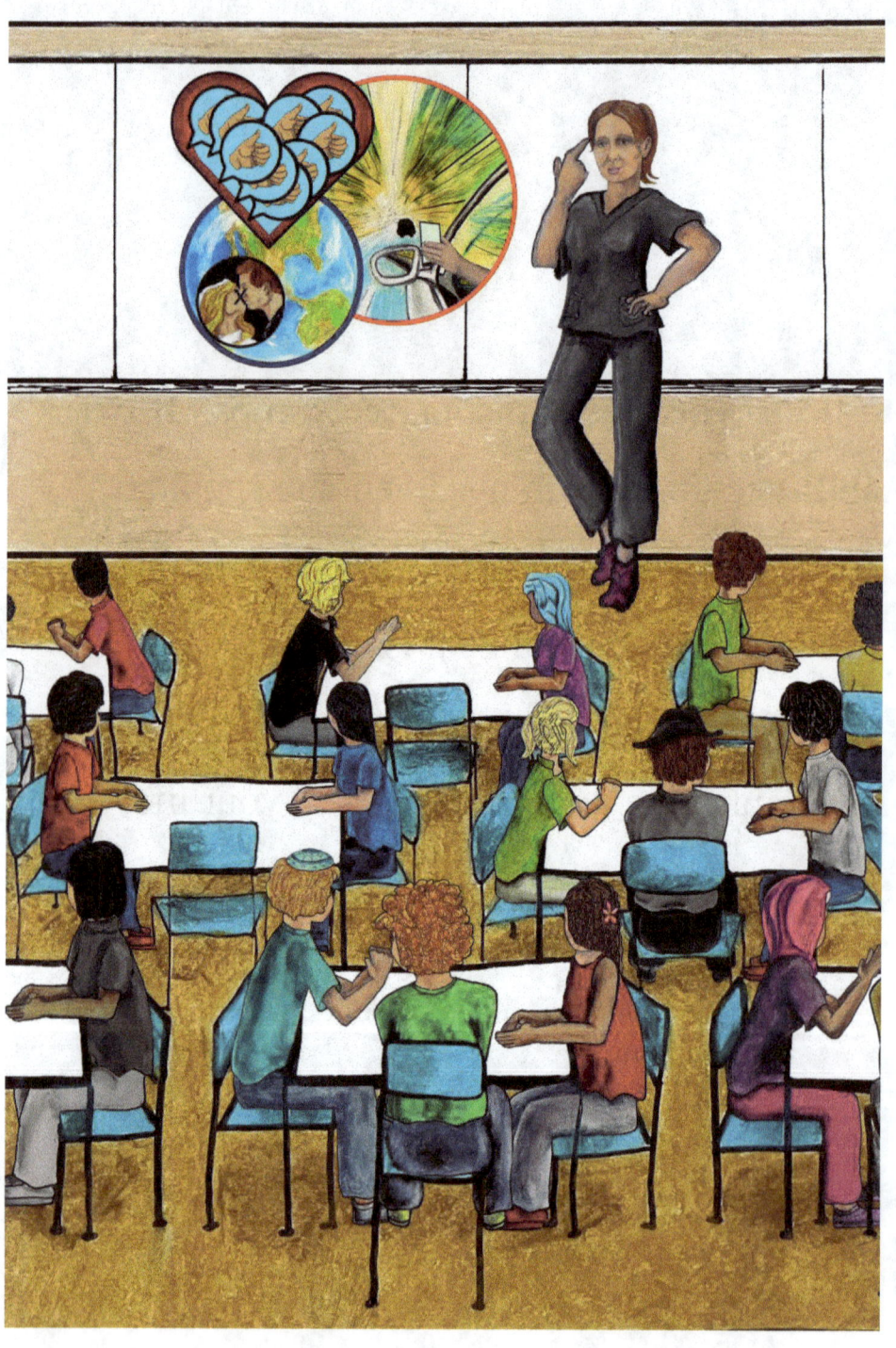

"If you use social media during dangerous situations like texting while driving, then you may be addicted. If you reduce the amount of real-world interactions you have so that you can use social media, then you may be addicted. If you start needing more and more likes for each post just to get the same amount of pleasure, then you may be addicted," says Nurse Dorothea.

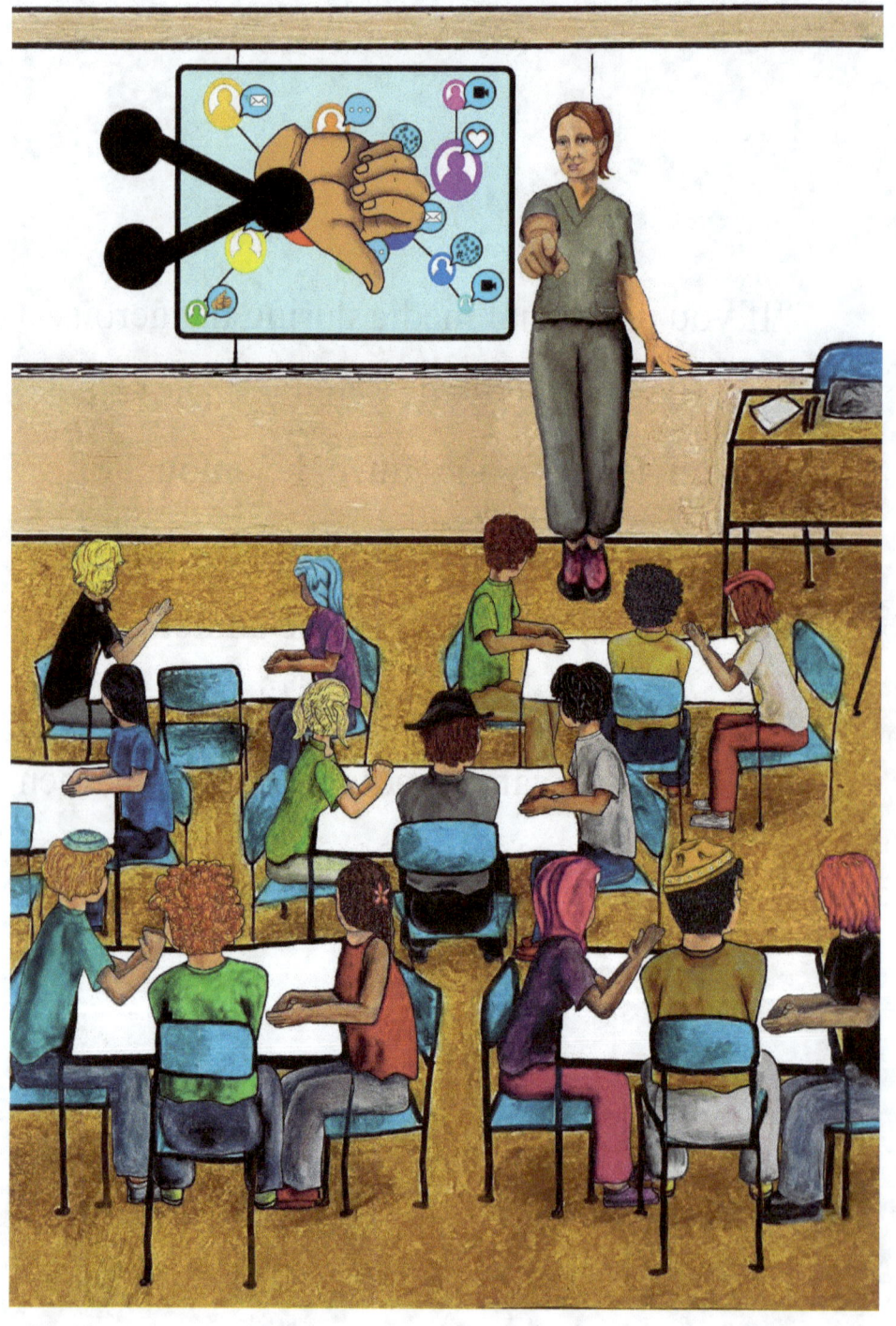

"We are going to continue our discussion on the negative effects of social media. Now, this time I would like all of you in the room, those watching the show and those reading the book, to think about something negative that you have experienced, done, or felt with social media. Share with those around you or write in your journal. Please take some time to do that now."

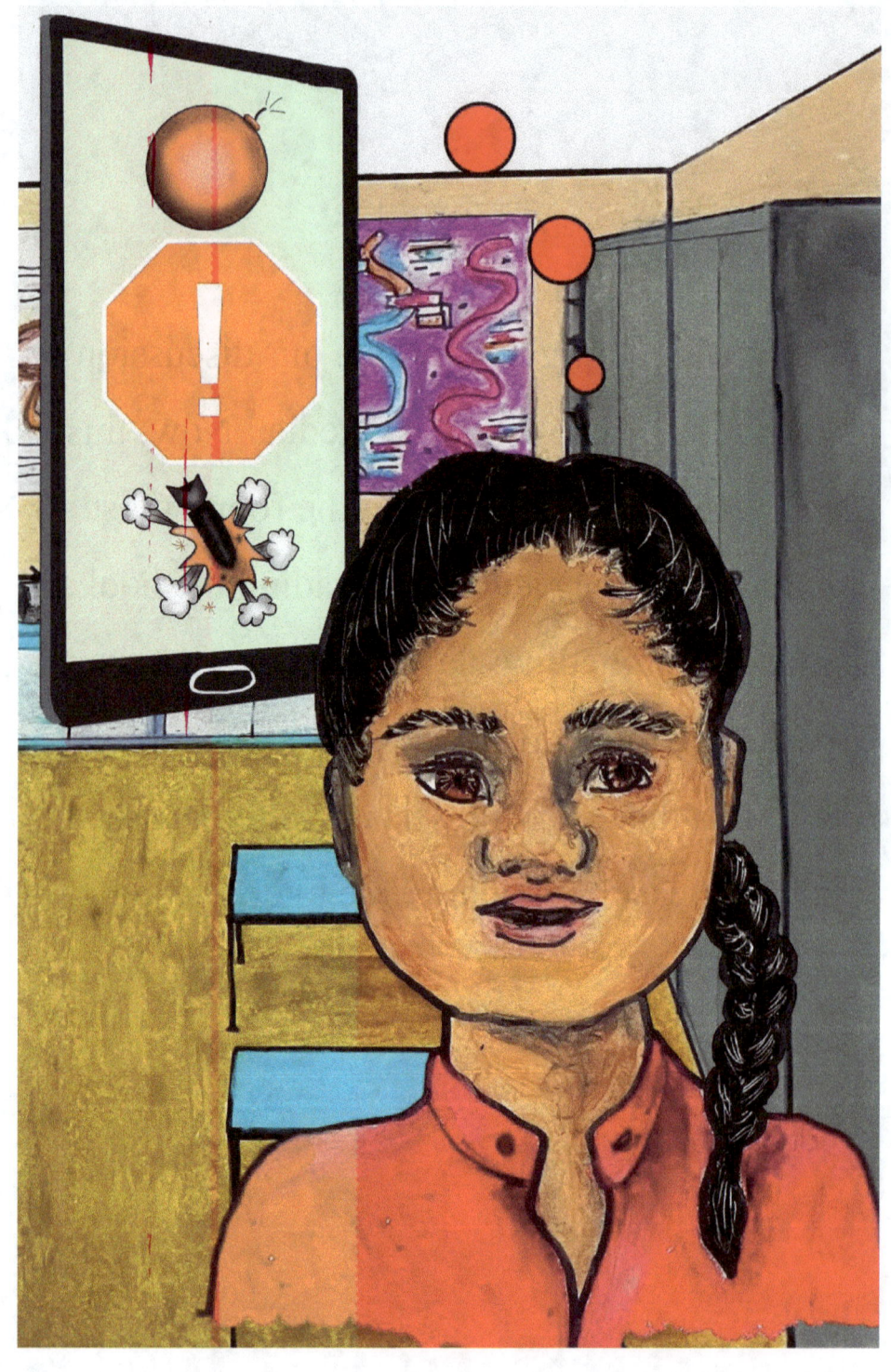

Pia raises her hand, and Nurse Dorothea calls on her to talk. "I have seen people harming themselves and some harming other people in some videos. Some of these videos still give me nightmares which affects my sleep and causes me to have a bad day the next morning."

"I'm sorry to hear that. That sounds really scary. Maybe this is something to bring up to your therapist or psychiatrist at your next visit," says Nurse Dorothea.

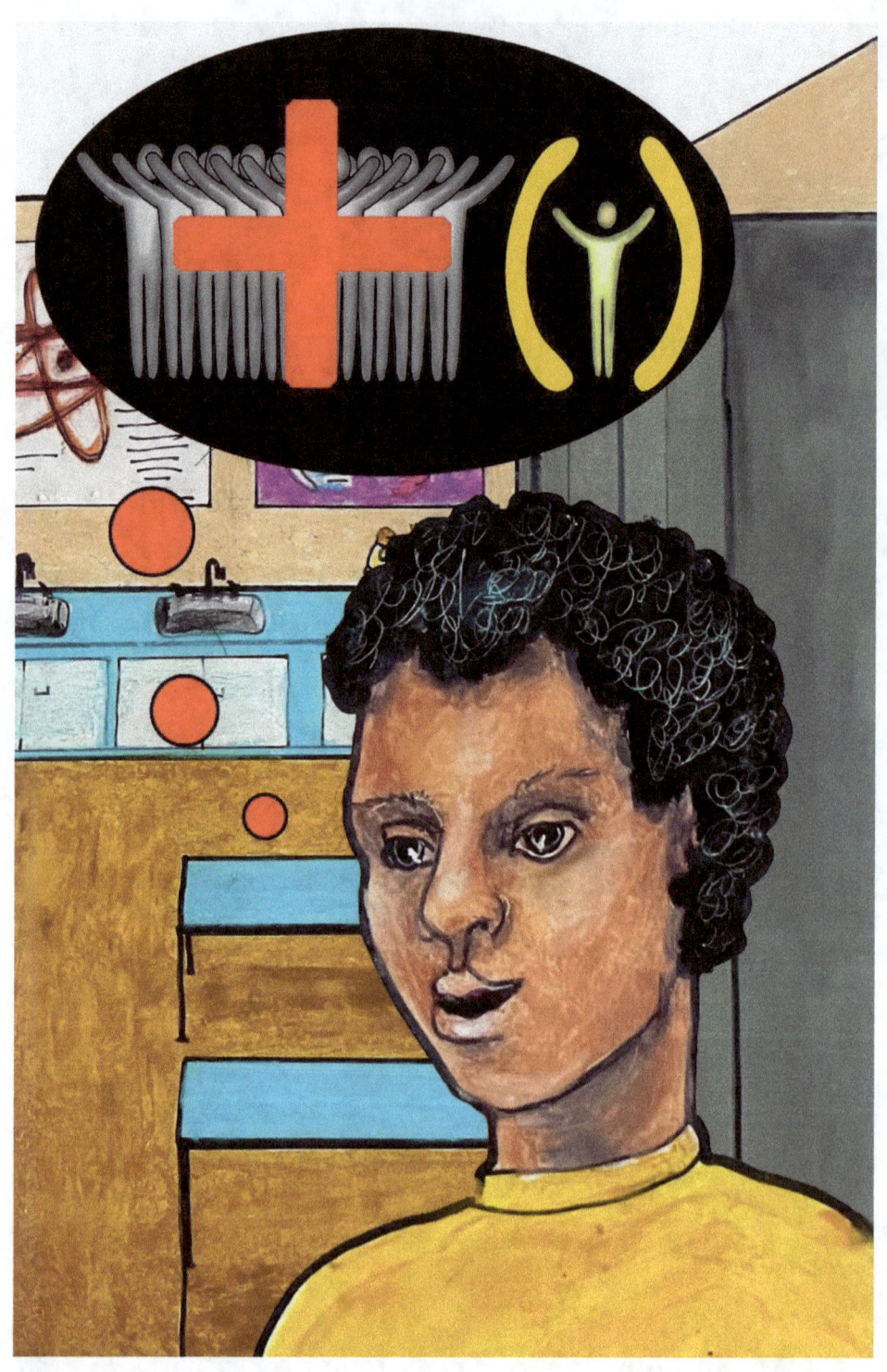

Ekon raises his hand, and Nurse Dorothea calls on him to talk. "After getting rejected on social media, I chose to isolate myself. I became very lonely and felt hopeless sometimes. I would come home and go straight to my room, listen to music, and avoid talking to my family. I felt they wouldn't understand, so I just kept my problems and my feelings to myself."

"We should all be careful about isolating ourselves. We are social beings and if we don't communicate with others about our fears, dreams, and feelings, then we can develop depression, etc.," says Nurse Dorothea.

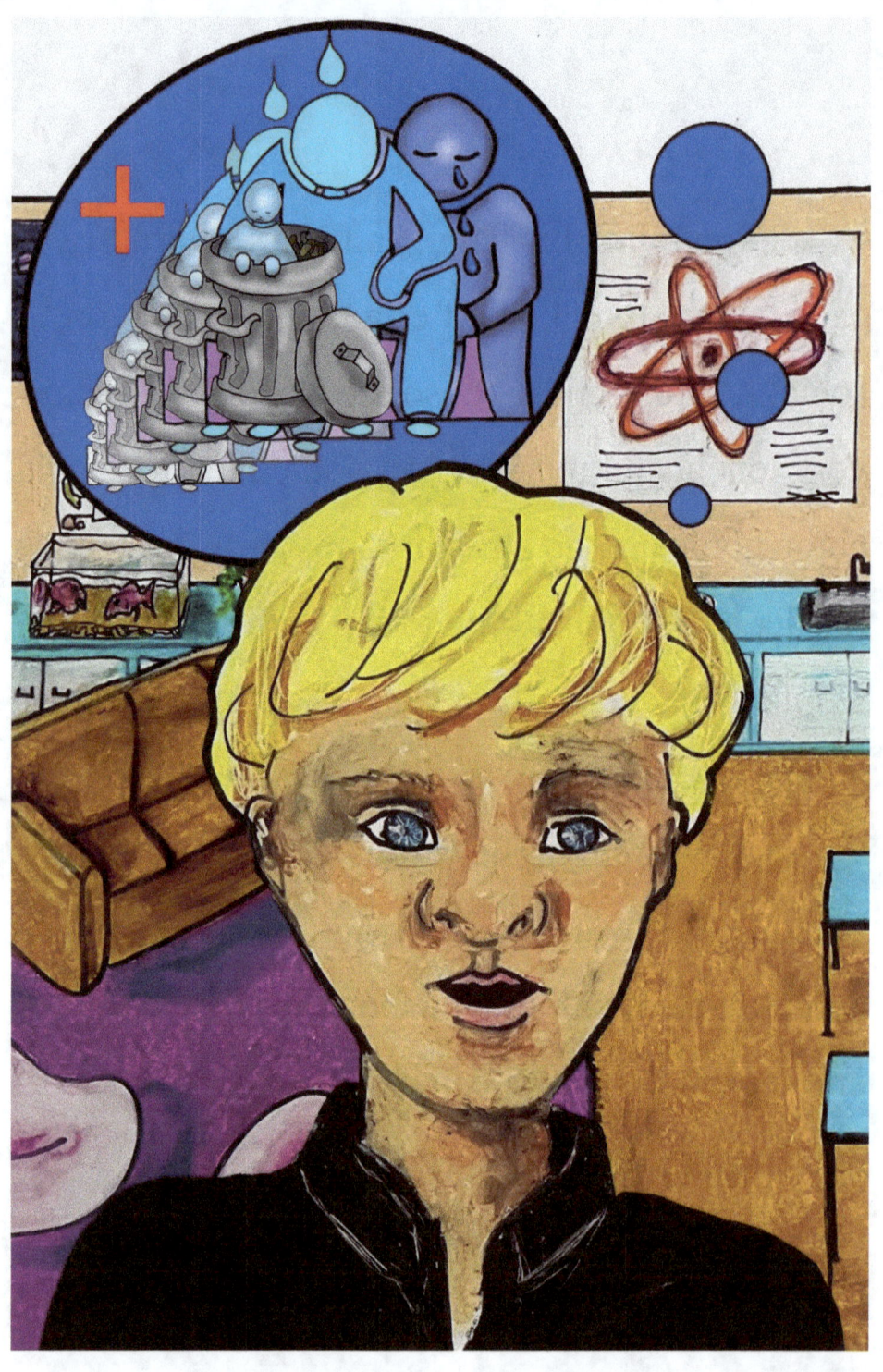

Dimitry raises his hand, and Nurse Dorothea calls on him to talk. "Some people said some mean things to me one time on social media and I took it really personal. I became depressed and my mom had me see a therapist."

"I'm sorry that you went through that, but that is great that you got some help. There are a lot of resources out there. We just need some help finding them," says Nurse Dorothea.

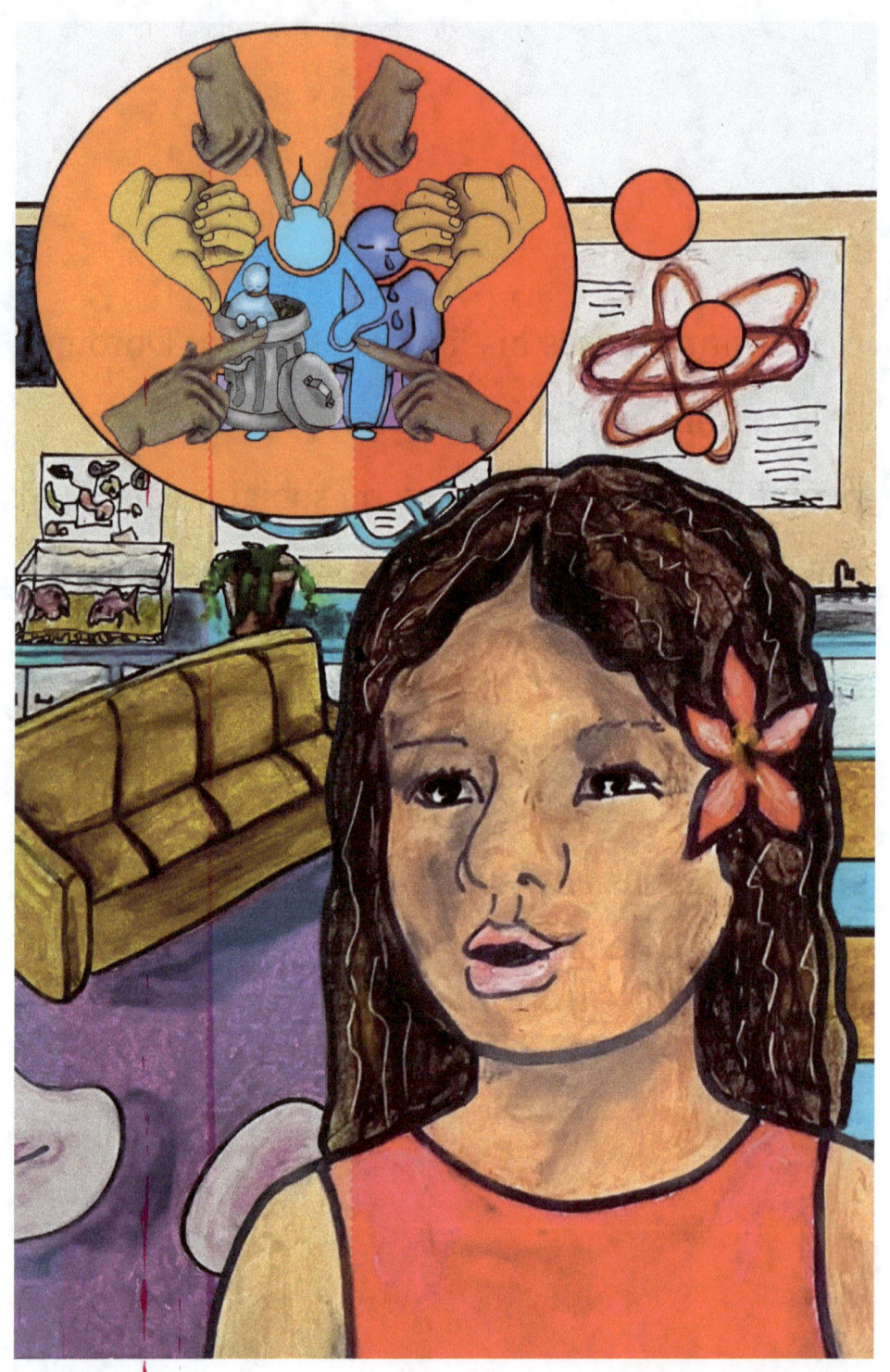

Kalani raises her hand, and Nurse Dorothea calls on her to talk. "I've been bullied online and have seen others get bullied. It used to make me sad and now it makes me angry. I don't like to feel angry like that towards others, but those people don't know how it affects people in the long run. They need to stop."

"Good insight that you recognized the change in your emotions. Sometimes, bad situations help us find out what we believe is important, and you obviously feel that respecting others is important," says Nurse Dorothea.

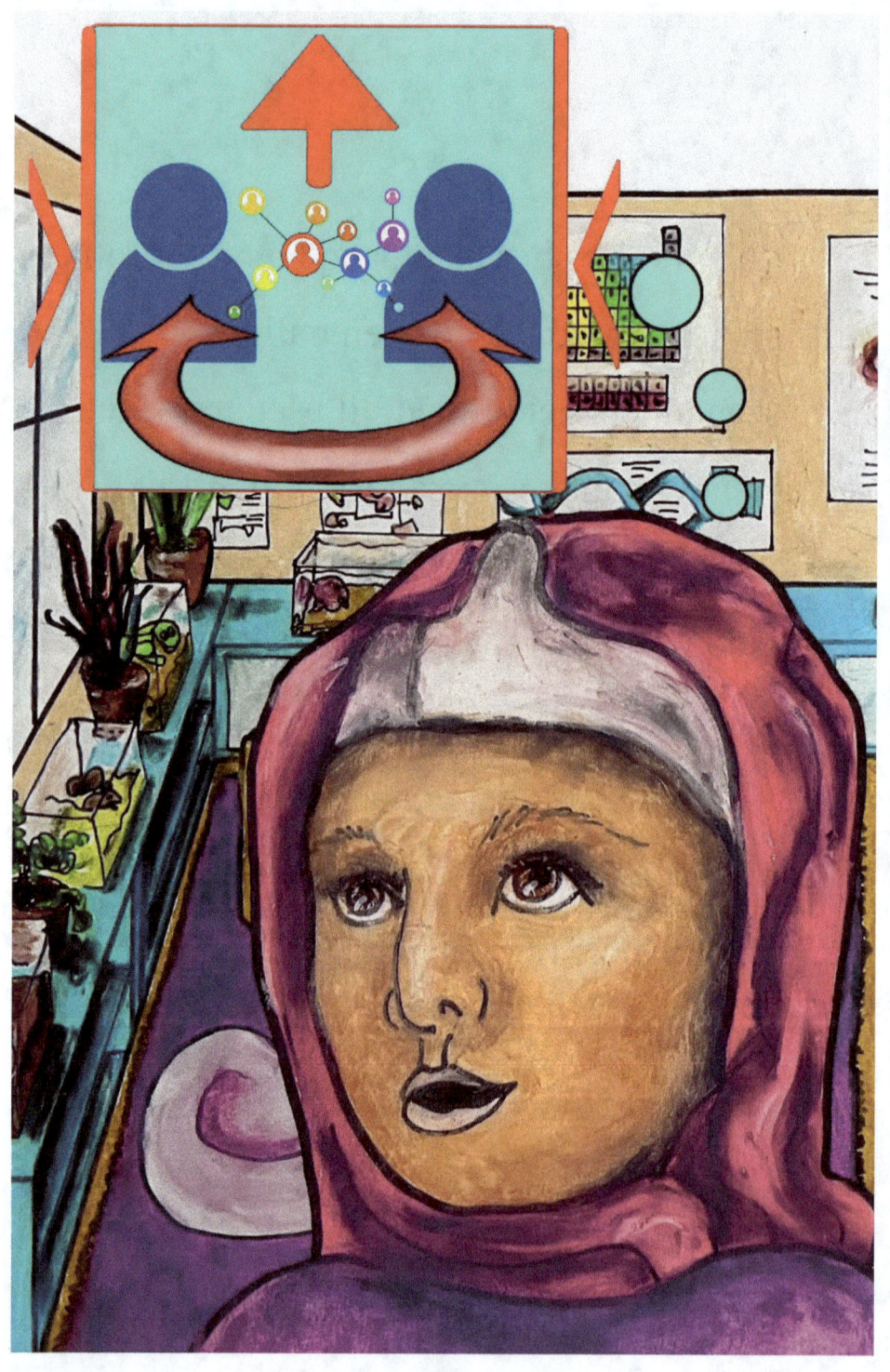

Fatima raises her hand, and Nurse Dorothea calls on her to talk. "I feel the need to compare myself to others. I feel the need to see how many likes I get with my posts and compare that to other people's posts. I feel bad sometimes when I get only a couple of likes or no comments while those around me get a lot of likes and a lot of comments."

"Social comparison can be a negative behavior pattern since it can cause some people to develop negative feelings when they think they are not equal to others," says Nurse Dorothea.

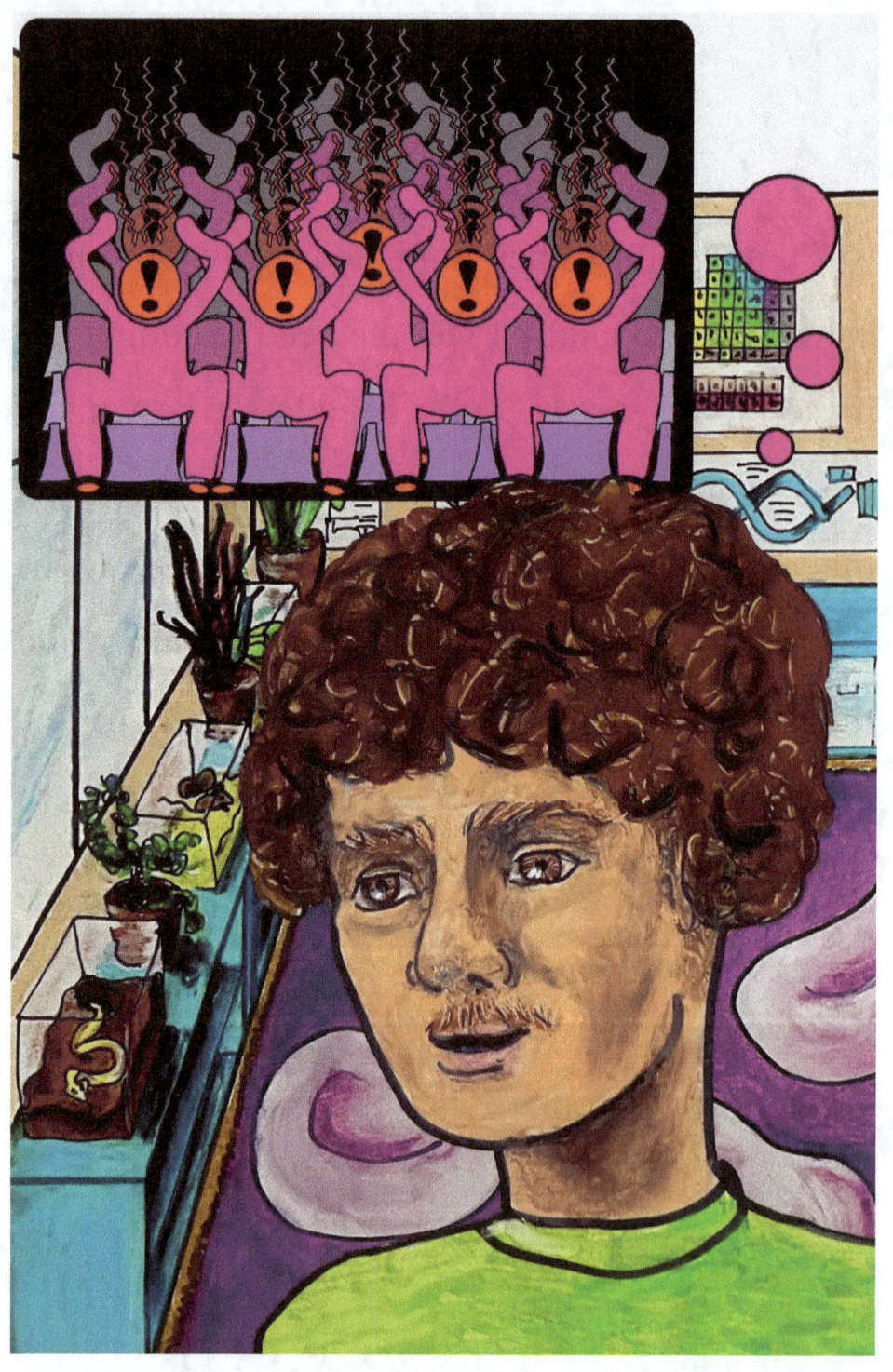

Gustavo raises his hand, and Nurse Dorothea calls on him to talk. "Some days, I feel more anxious when I am constantly checking my social media accounts. I wonder if I have a problem."

"Social media can become addictive for some, and some people may need to unplug and get off social media for a period of time to reset their feelings," says Nurse Dorothea.

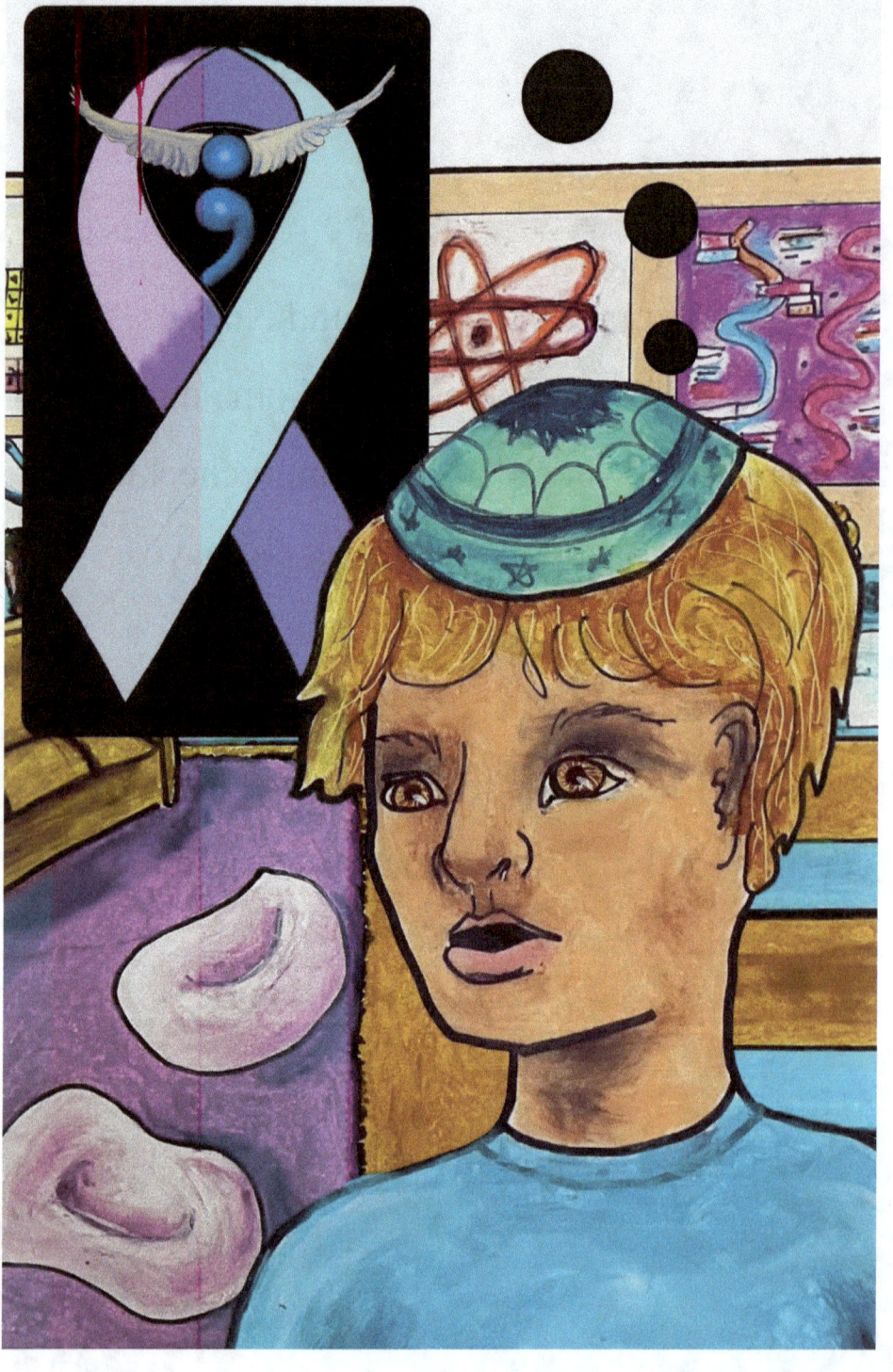

Levi raises his hand, and Nurse Dorothea calls on him to talk. "A friend told me once that after using social media constantly for weeks, he started feeling suicidal and wanted his life to end because of bullying and seeing dark things on the internet."

"Some people who are vulnerable to suicidal thinking can have problems when they used social media, especially when they are exposed to negative images and words. We need a strong social support system so that we are buffered from the negative effects of social media. If you feel that you are being cyberbullied, seek help from a trusted adult," says Nurse Dorothea.

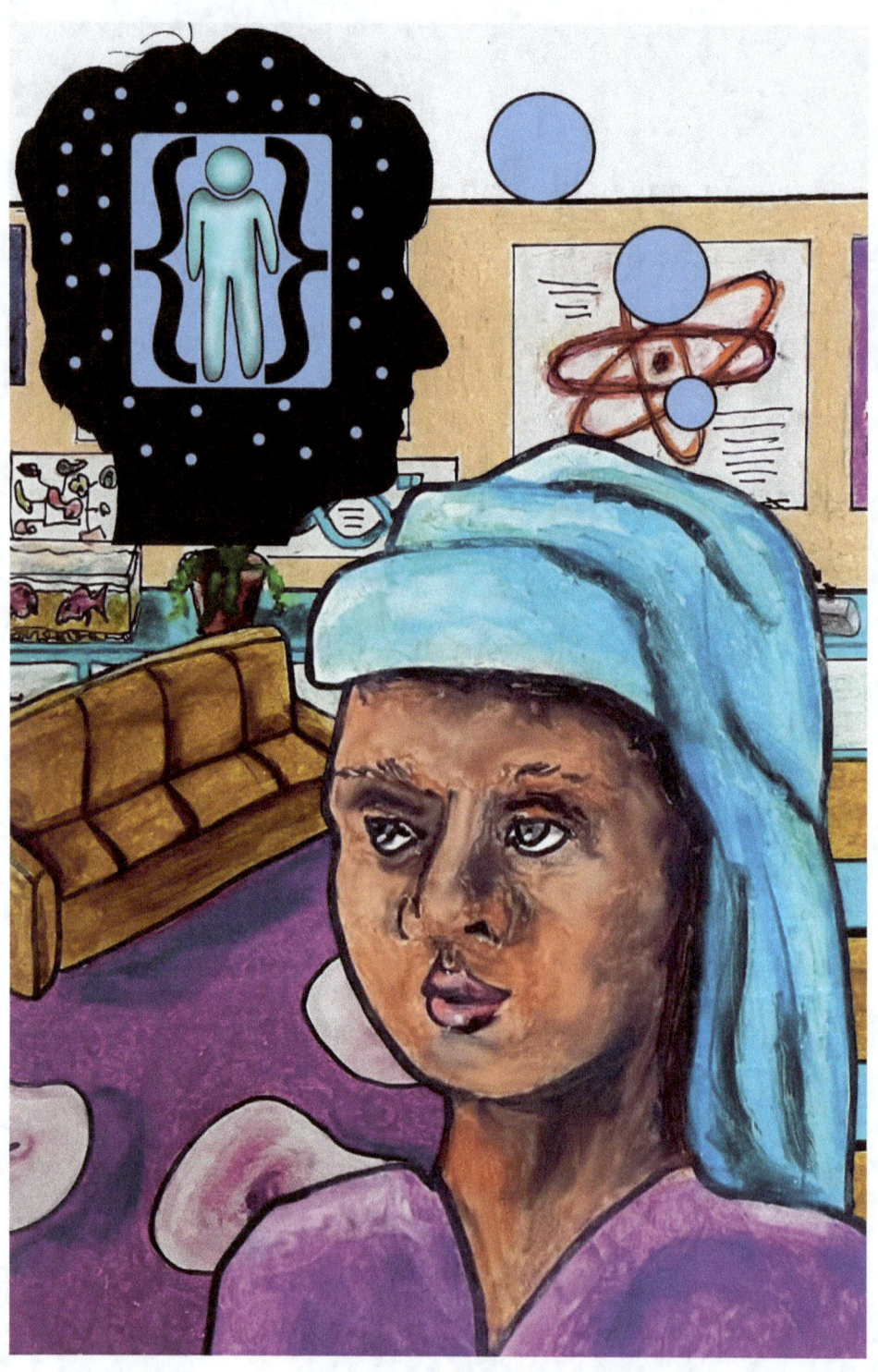

Yuliana raises her hand, and Nurse Dorothea calls on her to talk. "I've experienced greater feelings of loneliness with social media at times. I know some people talk about how they feel supported when they have a social group online that they are a part of, but there have been times that I felt like I was very lonely and didn't have purpose."

"You bring up an interesting connection. When we feel lonely, we should seek to discover our purpose in life. Purpose can help our mental health in many ways, so if you feel you don't have any, use that as motivation to try to discover your purpose," says Nurse Dorothea.

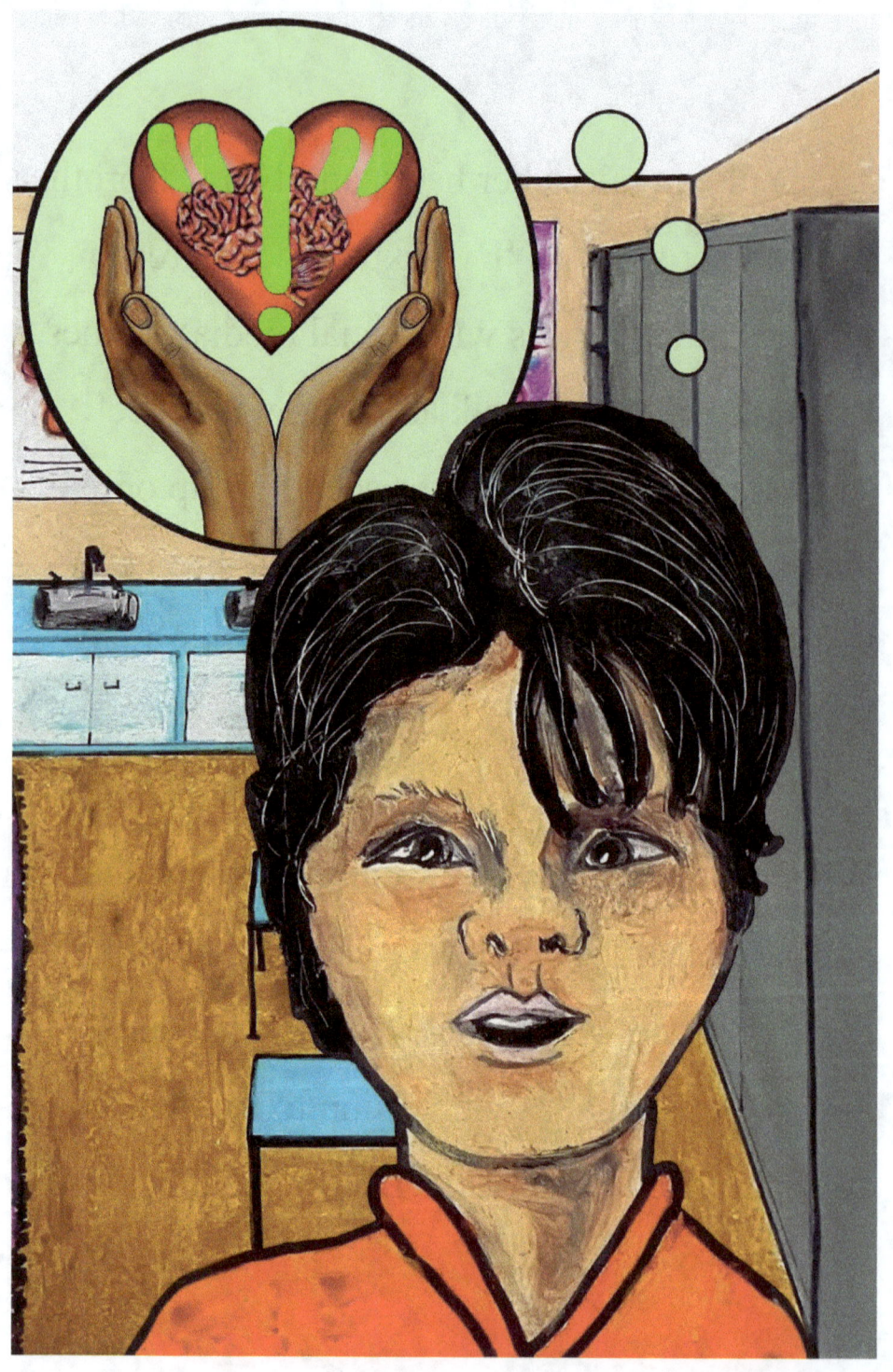

Kenji raises his hand, and Nurse Dorothea calls on him to talk. "I've seen that some people have their mental health symptoms worsen from too much social media use. I've seen them become sadder and more anxious. It makes me sad to see my friends sad, and I don't think I have enough tools to help them."

"We should use social media in moderation like most things in life. I'm glad you are attending this after-school club so that you can get more tools to not only help yourself but also your loved ones in your life," says Nurse Dorothea.

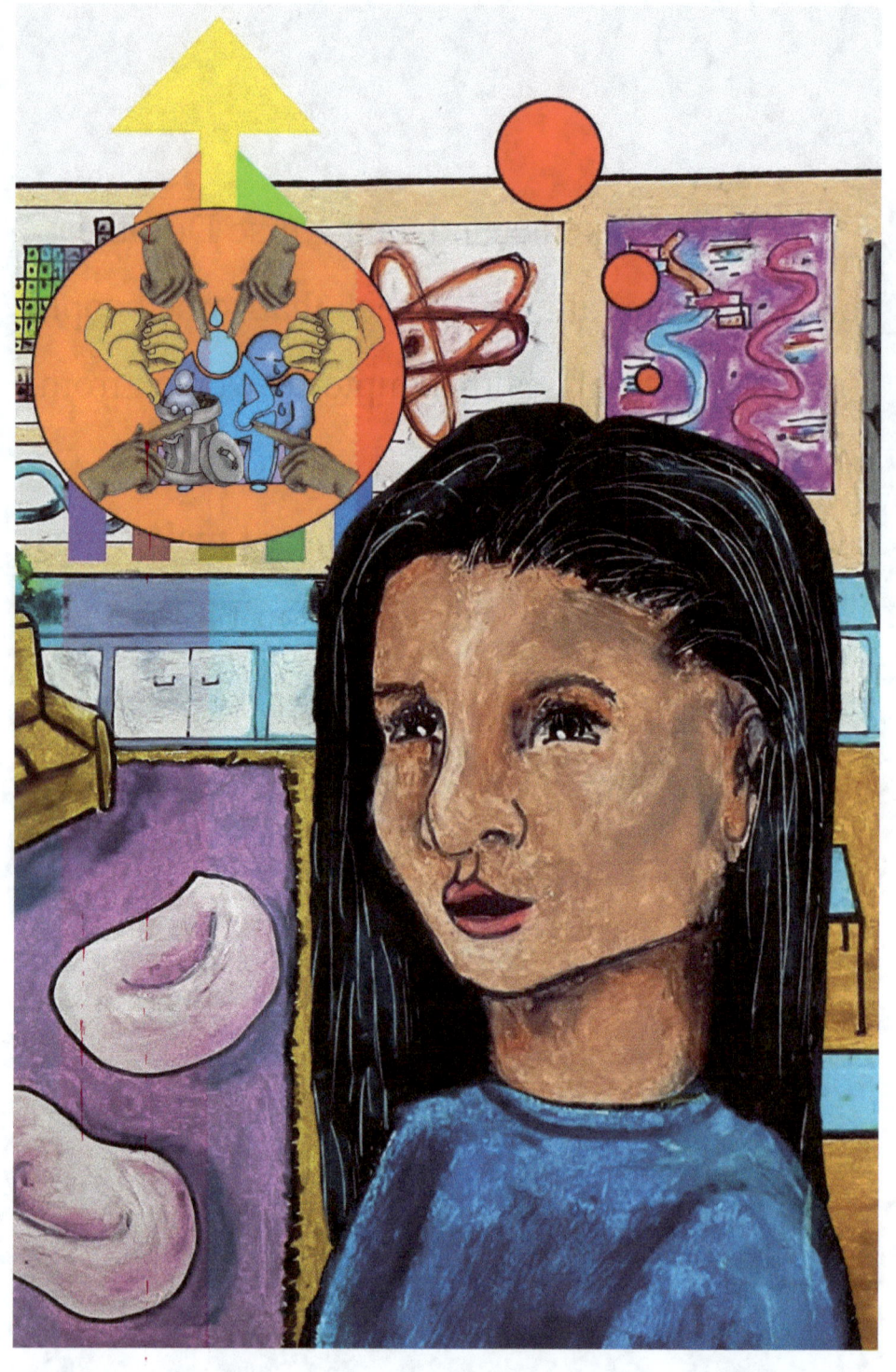

Diwa raises her hand, and Nurse Dorothea calls on her to talk. "I think some people who are depressed are at increased risk of bullying when they get online. Some people are mean, and they want to make others feel bad."

"Since we don't always know other people's intentions, we should avoid assuming we know what other people think. It is true that some people in the world say and do mean things to others. Some people may have disorders and need assistance to recognize proper cultural speech and behaviors. We need to be good role models and demonstrate civility. People who act with incivility may be involved with law enforcement in the future," says Nurse Dorothea.

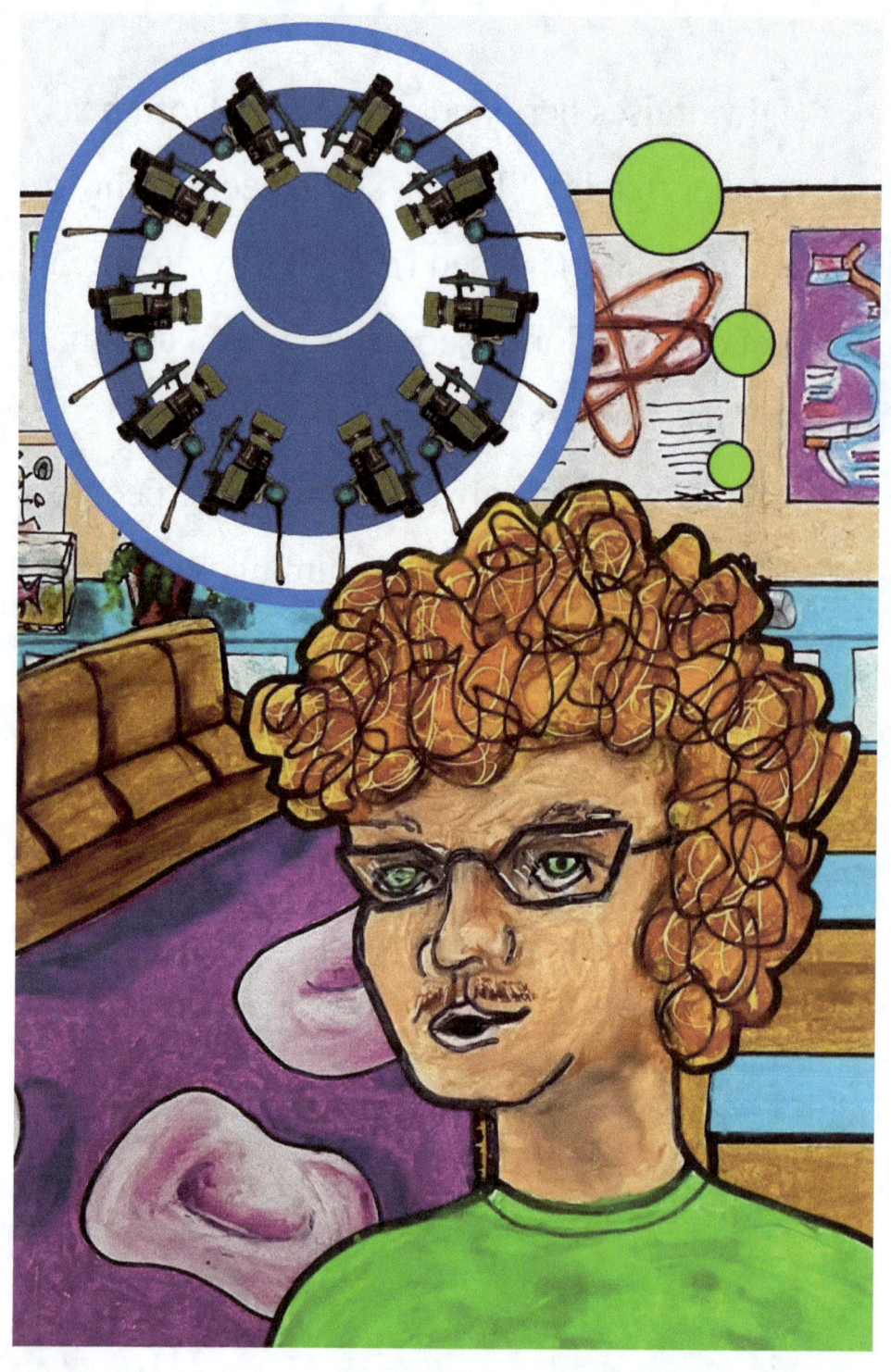

Connor raises his hand, and Nurse Dorothea calls on him to talk. "Social media can be used to violate people's privacy. I'm a private person and don't want the world to know lots of things about me. Since we must create user profiles for social media, I've decided to use social media very little."

"Privacy is very important to many. Also, talking about privacy, make sure you review your privacy settings regularly on all your media accounts," says Nurse Dorothea.

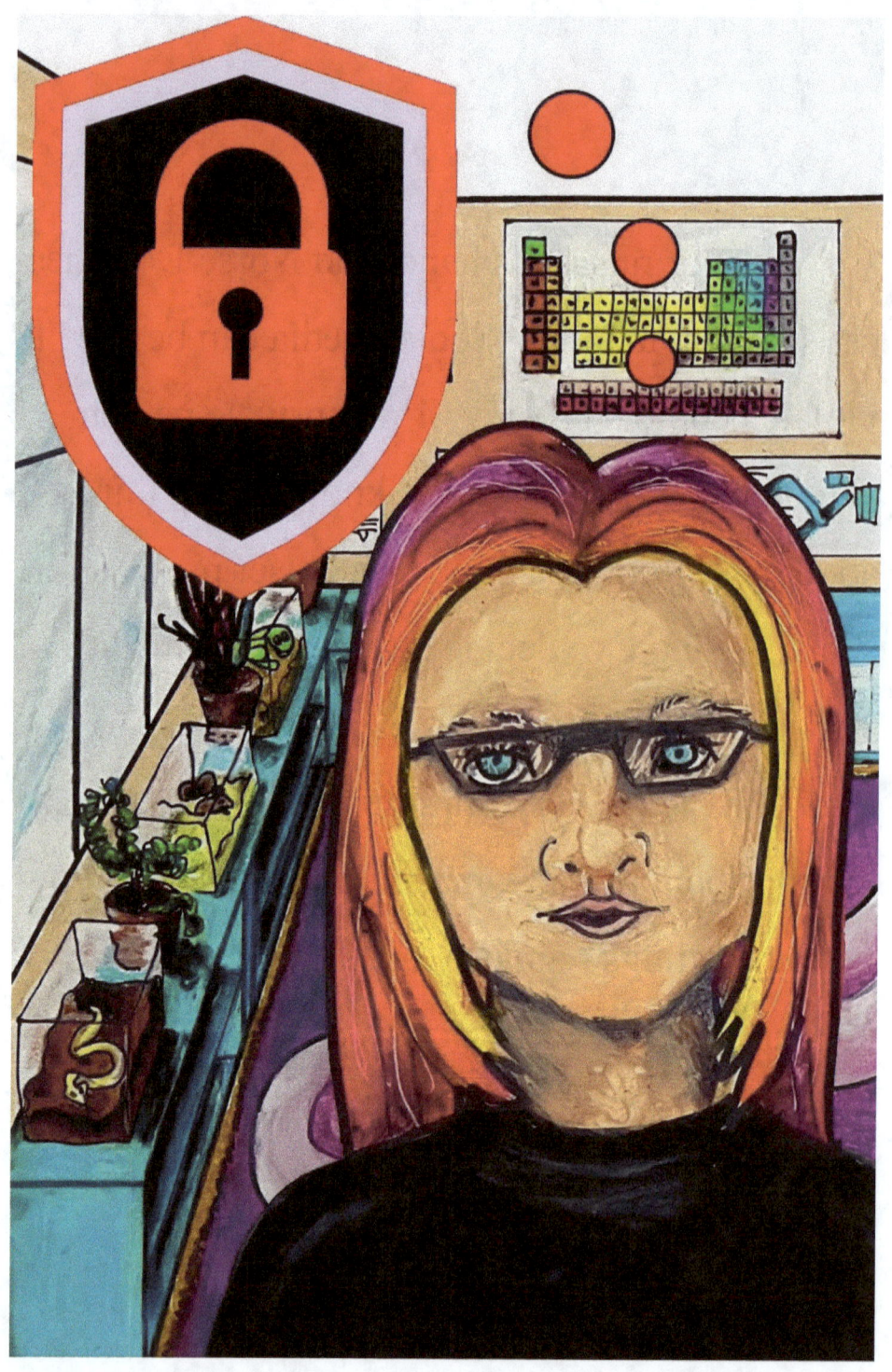

Juniper raises her hand, and Nurse Dorothea calls on her to talk. "Along the same lines, confidentiality can be violated on social media. Once, I texted something personal to someone I thought was a friend and then they took a screenshot of the text and posted it on social media for everyone to see what I was dealing with. I thought what I texted would stay confidential."

"Once things are in the digital world, it is very hard to remove it, and sometimes it is impossible due to all the sharing. Be very careful of what photos you take, what text messages you write, and what videos you record of yourself, even if it is doing something silly. Also, do not share passwords to your social media accounts with your friends, since they may cancel your account if there is a bad break-up," says Nurse Dorothea.

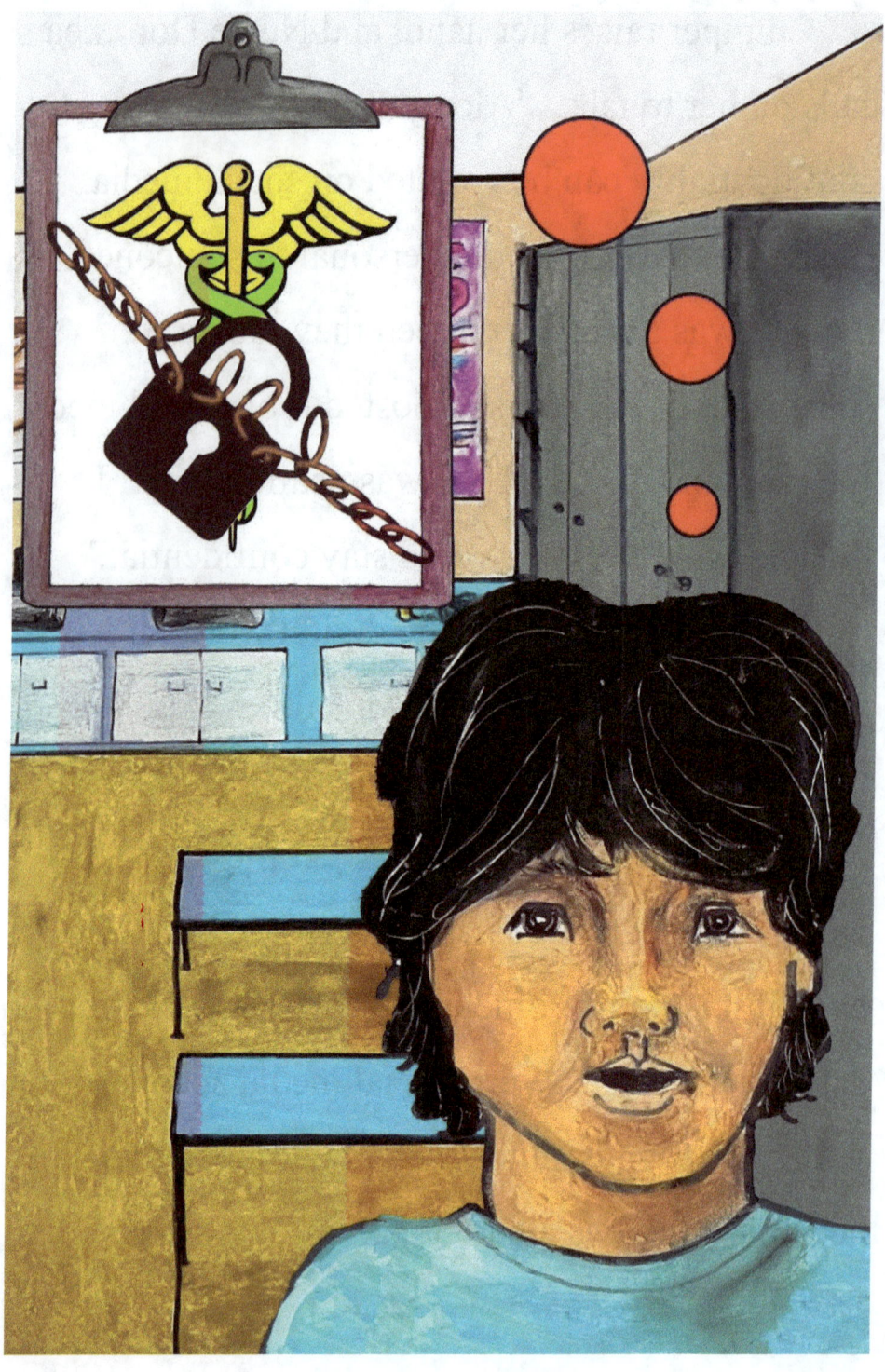

Ji Ho raises his hand, and Nurse Dorothea calls on him to talk. "Also, regarding confidentiality, I've seen some people's personal health information get disclosed on social media. Now, everyone knows about their illness. It seems like it is embarrassing for some people to have that information shared so freely."

"There are laws against disclosing other people's health information, so it is best to not say anything and not share gossip. Only disclose other people's health information if you are medical provider and then, do it only with people you have permission to disclose it to. Also, never share naked pictures of yourself. They could end up on the cloud forever. You could get charged with child pornography if you are a minor," says Nurse Dorothea.

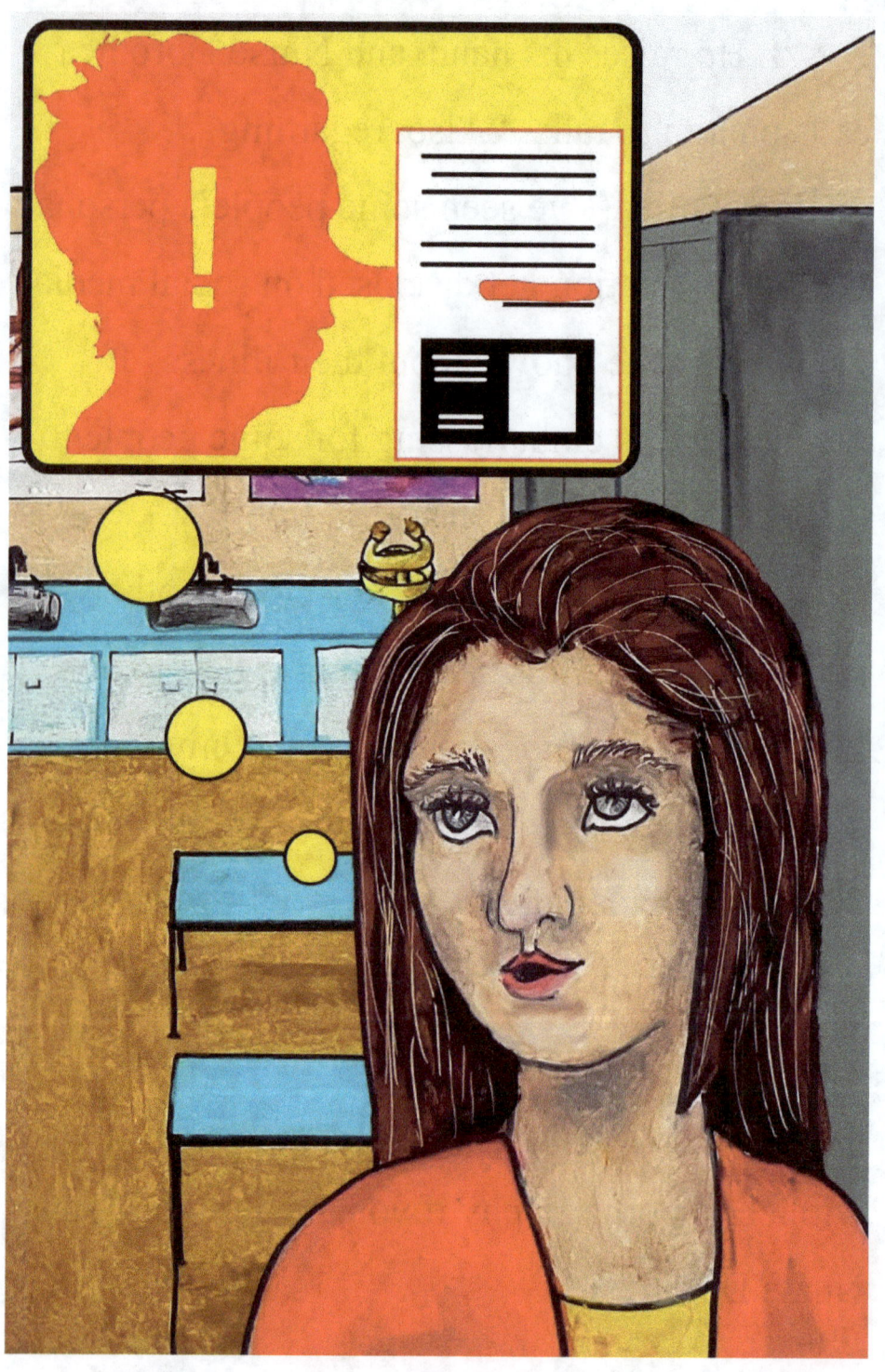

Awira raises her hand, and Nurse Dorothea calls on her to talk. "Social media can be used to share misleading information. This can cause people to make bad choices which could affect the rest of their lives."

"Misleading info can harm others so be careful to share only what is researched and true to the best of your knowledge. If you don't know, then it probably shouldn't be shared," says Nurse Dorothea.

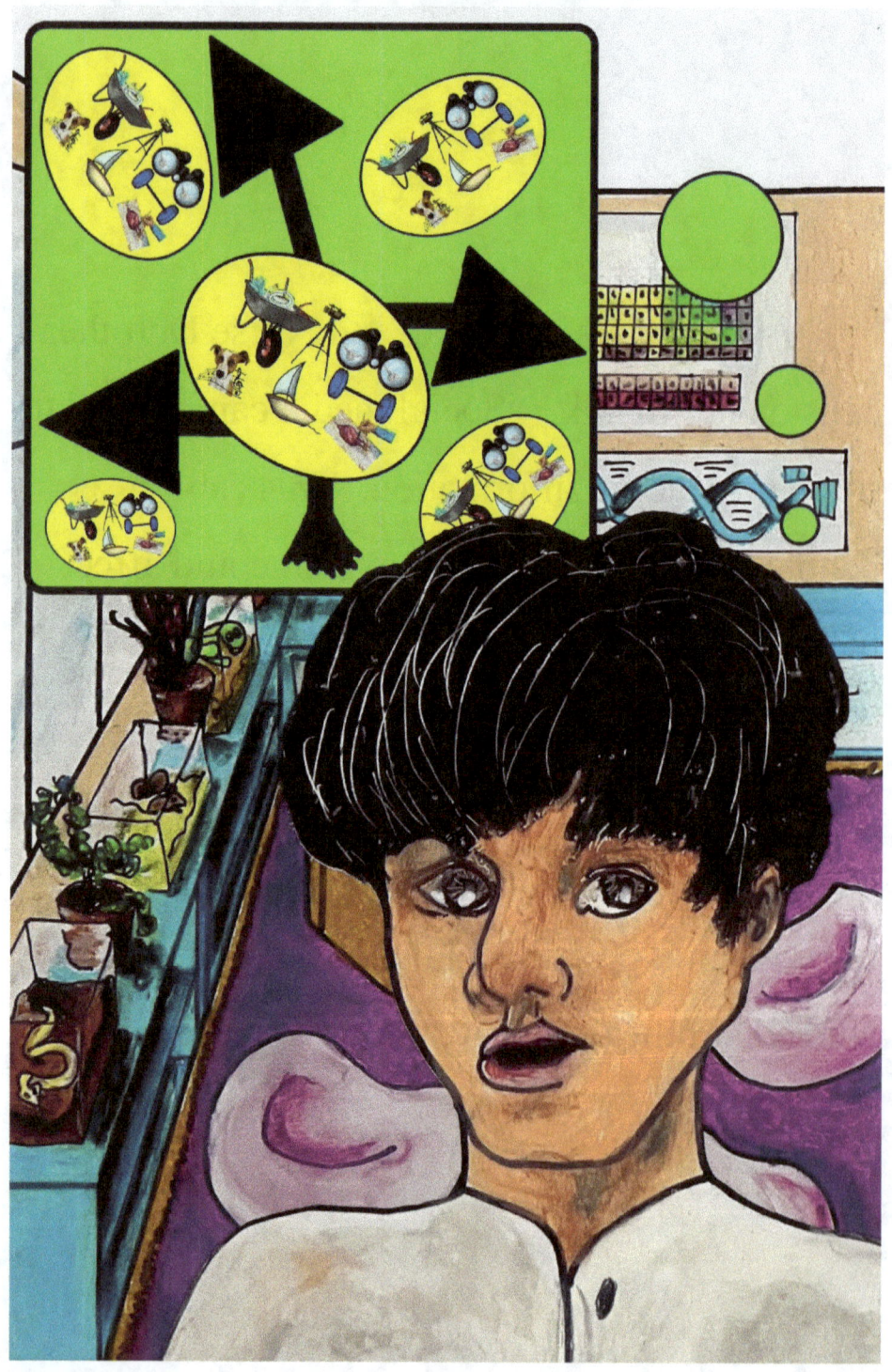

Antonio raises his hand, and Nurse Dorothea calls on him to talk. "There have been groups of people online pressuring me to try marijuana, and I did. I regret it now because it caused some hallucinations that were scary. I think the marijuana may have been laced with something. Pressure by the group made me make a poor choice."

"Thanks for sharing your experience," says Nurse Dorothea.

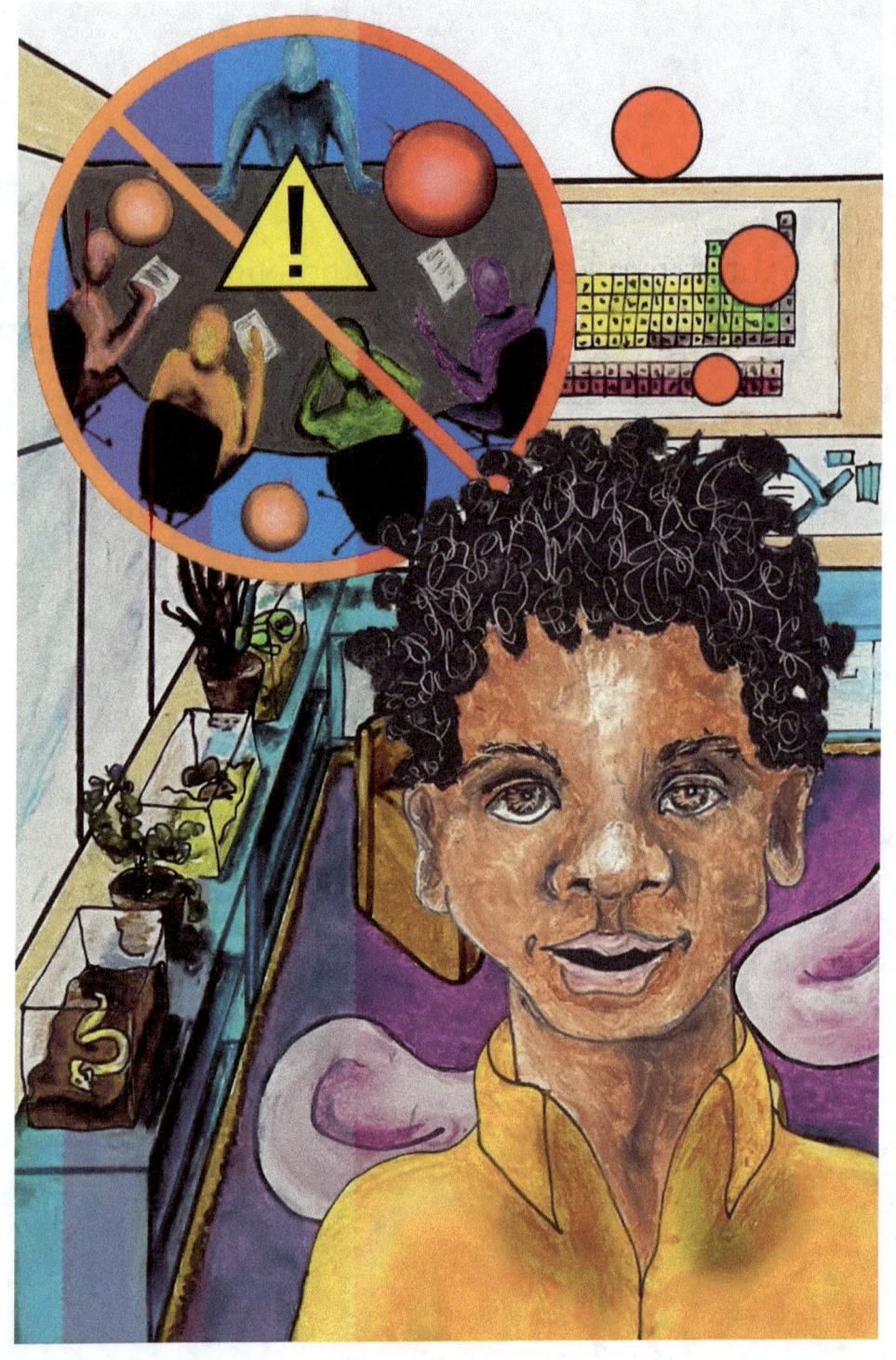

Amari raises his hand, and Nurse Dorothea calls on him to talk. "I've seen some people on message boards make threats to others about their employment saying they would find out where they worked and try to get them fired. That's not right."

"Employment is an important part of people's lives since, as adults, we spend so much of our waking hours at work. Threats to employment are not funny," says Nurse Dorothea.

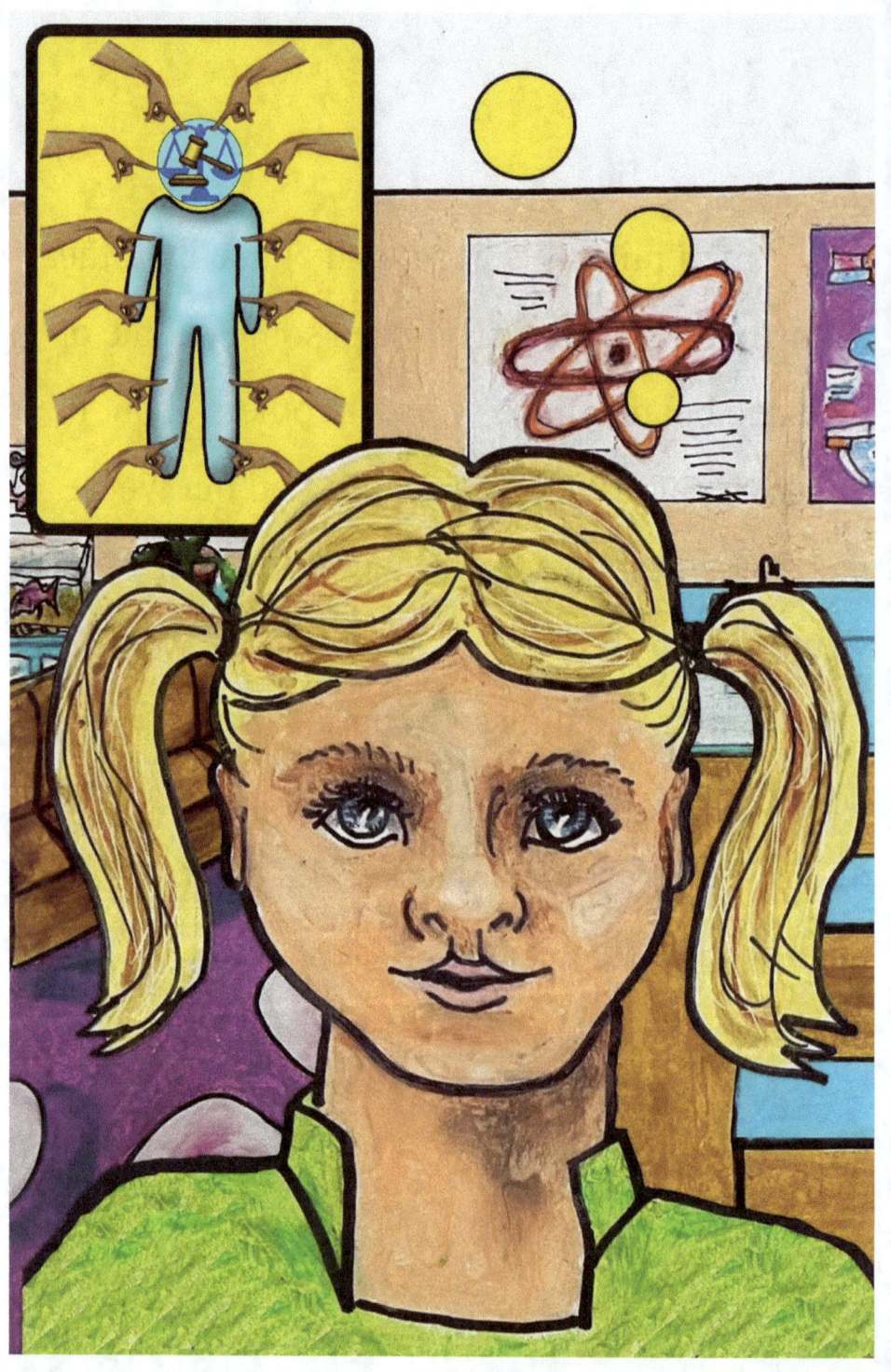

Frida raises her hand, and Nurse Dorothea calls on her to talk. "There have been times that I was singled out and judged about something. I didn't like that feeling that others were judging me and making me feel wrong."

"Stigma is an obstacle in most cultures that many different groups of people must deal with. We need to learn to stop producing stigma as a society," says Nurse Dorothea.

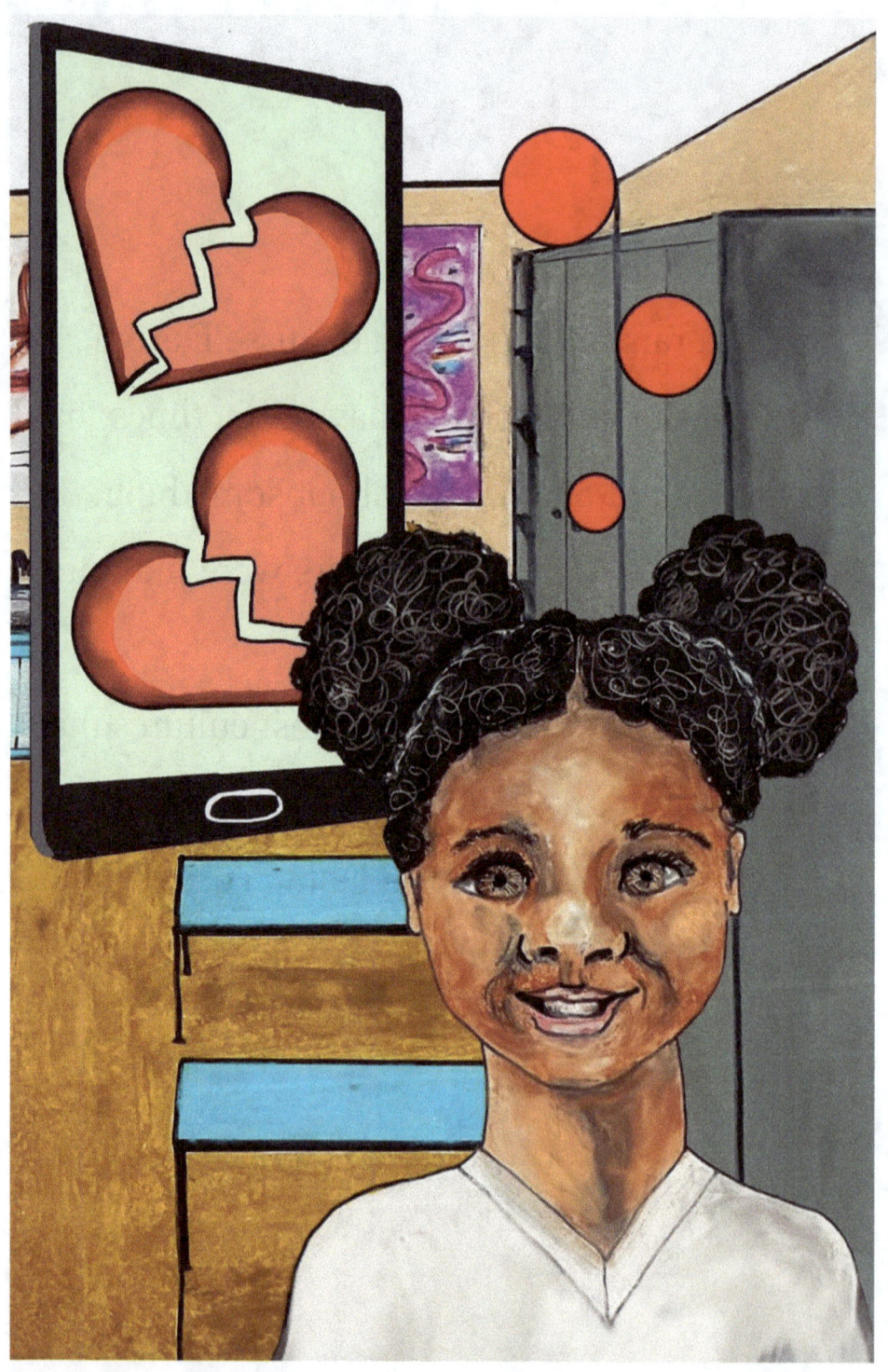

Amisha raises her hand, and Nurse Dorothea calls on her to talk. "I've seen social media interactions cause some people to break up their friendships with others as well as relationships with their partner. Breakups are hard. I've also seen some people pressure their partners into giving them their passwords for social media, and that doesn't seem right since we should have a right to privacy."

"You're right that sometimes the wrong thing is said or even something is perceived as wrong or mean. The other person may have a hard time seeing if it was the intention of the partner to cause relationship difficulties so the relationship may be broken. We need to respect each other's boundaries and give each other privacy," says Nurse Dorothea.

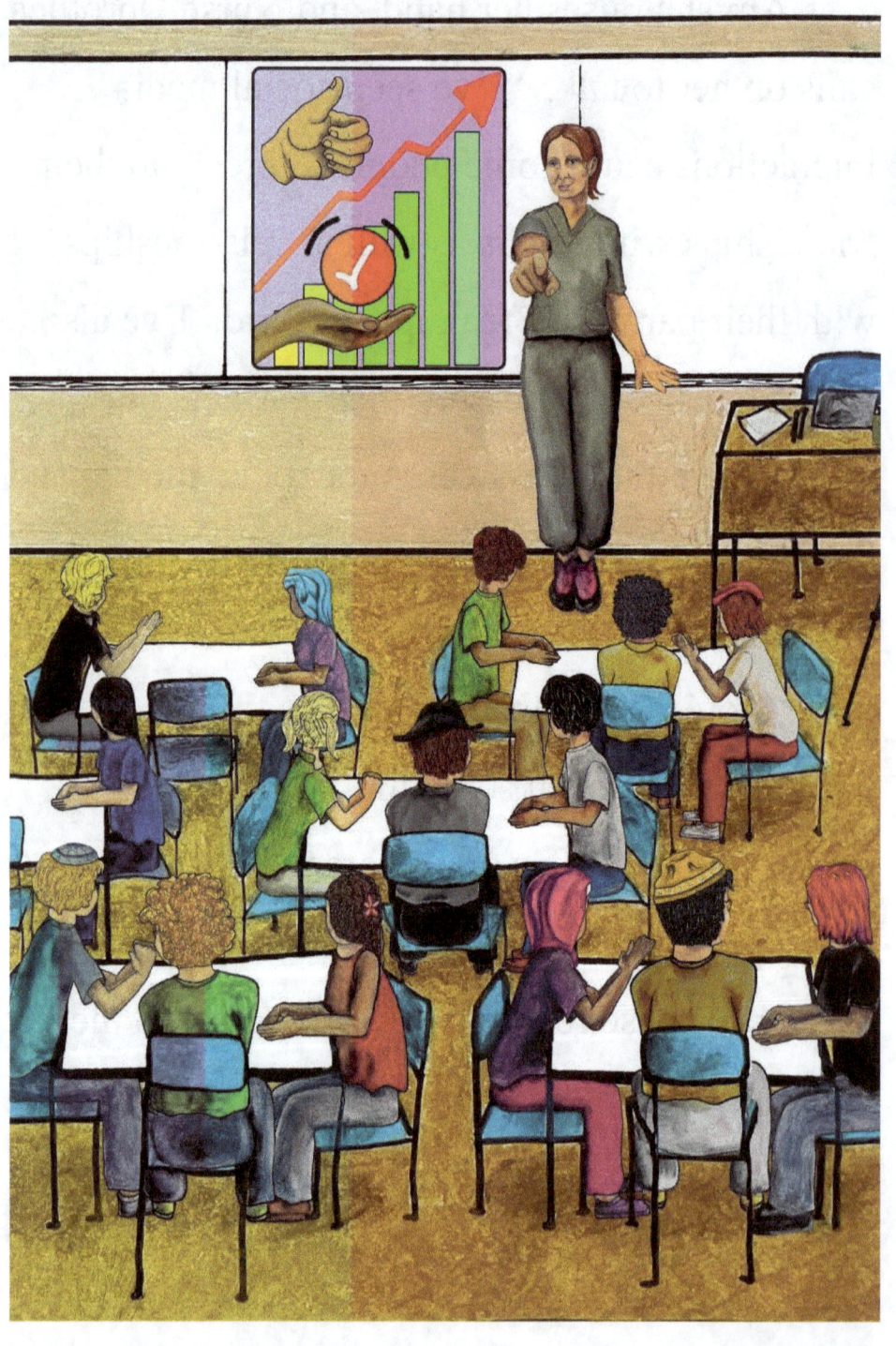

"Now that we have discussed the benefits and disadvantages of social media, let's discuss some things that you need to do or be aware of so that we can enjoy the benefits more often and the disadvantages less often."

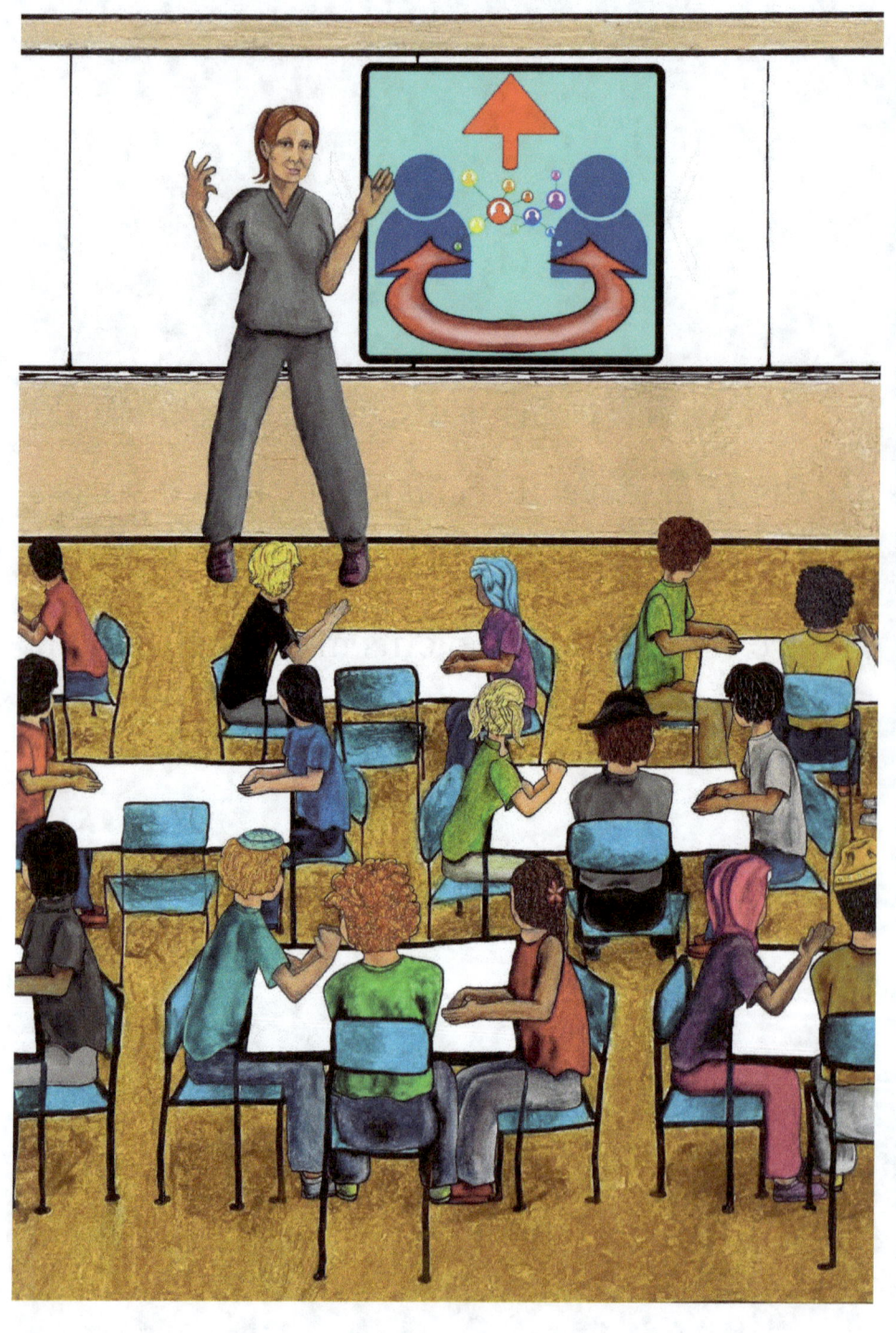

"You should learn to manage social comparison. This is a source of a lot of frustration and negative feelings people may have with social media. Learn to reframe your social comparison. For instance, maybe you only received 3 likes on your post because the content was not interesting to many people on your feed. Maybe you should set a smaller goal like having five likes per post instead of 100. Try to not compare yourself to others since we are unique, and the things we do help define who we are. You are not defined by someone else's success or failure. Post things in order to share instead of posting for likes. If you find yourself focusing on likes, maybe you should take a break from social media."

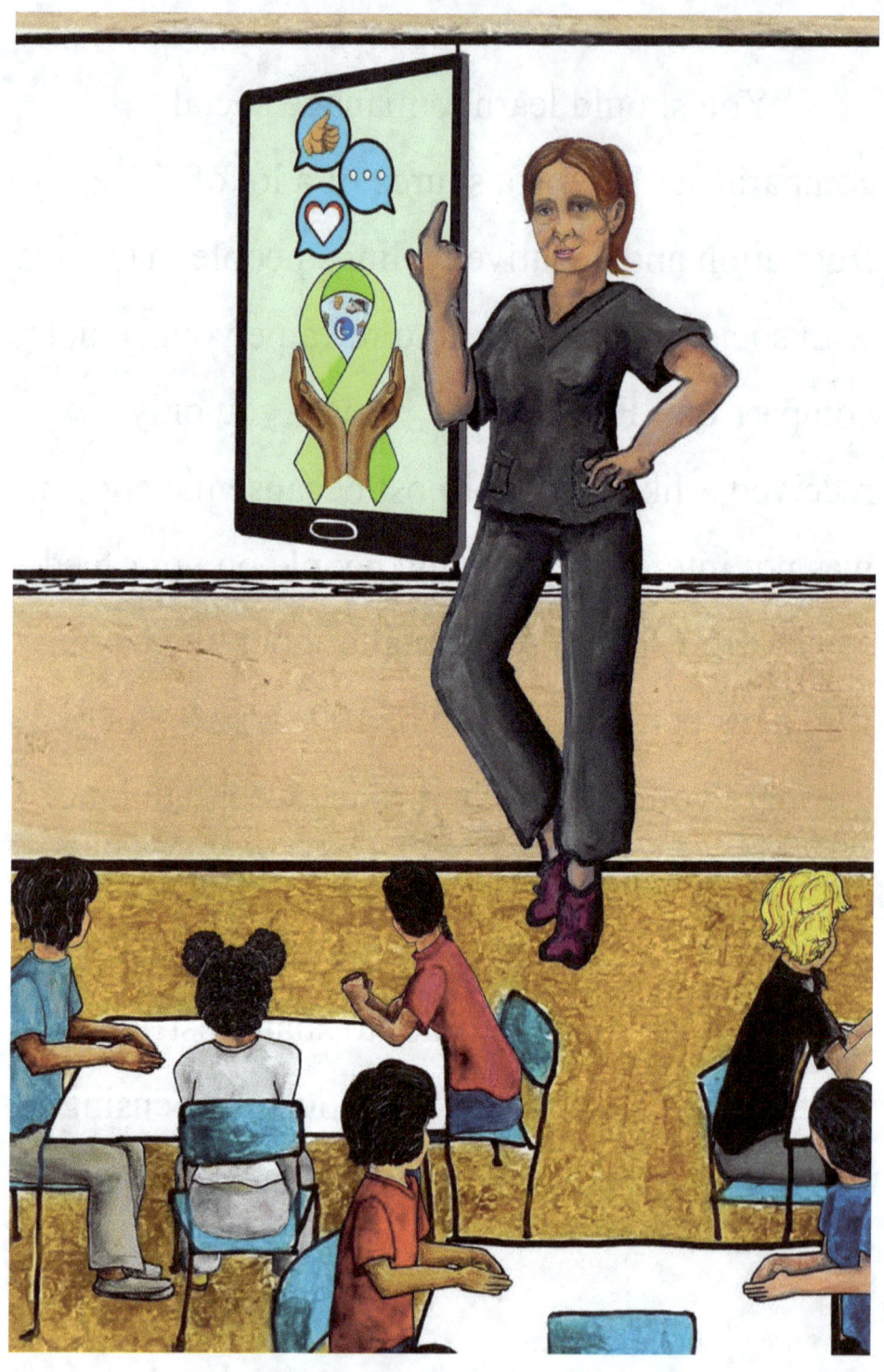

"We should learn how social media affects psychological needs. Maslow's hierarchy shows that after safety is secured in our lives, we will seek to belong. Social media helps us meet that psychological need of belonging. Embrace it, but also try to find other ways to belong instead of only using online tools. Have diversity in your psychological support. Use all the tools this world has to offer, not just an easy online method."

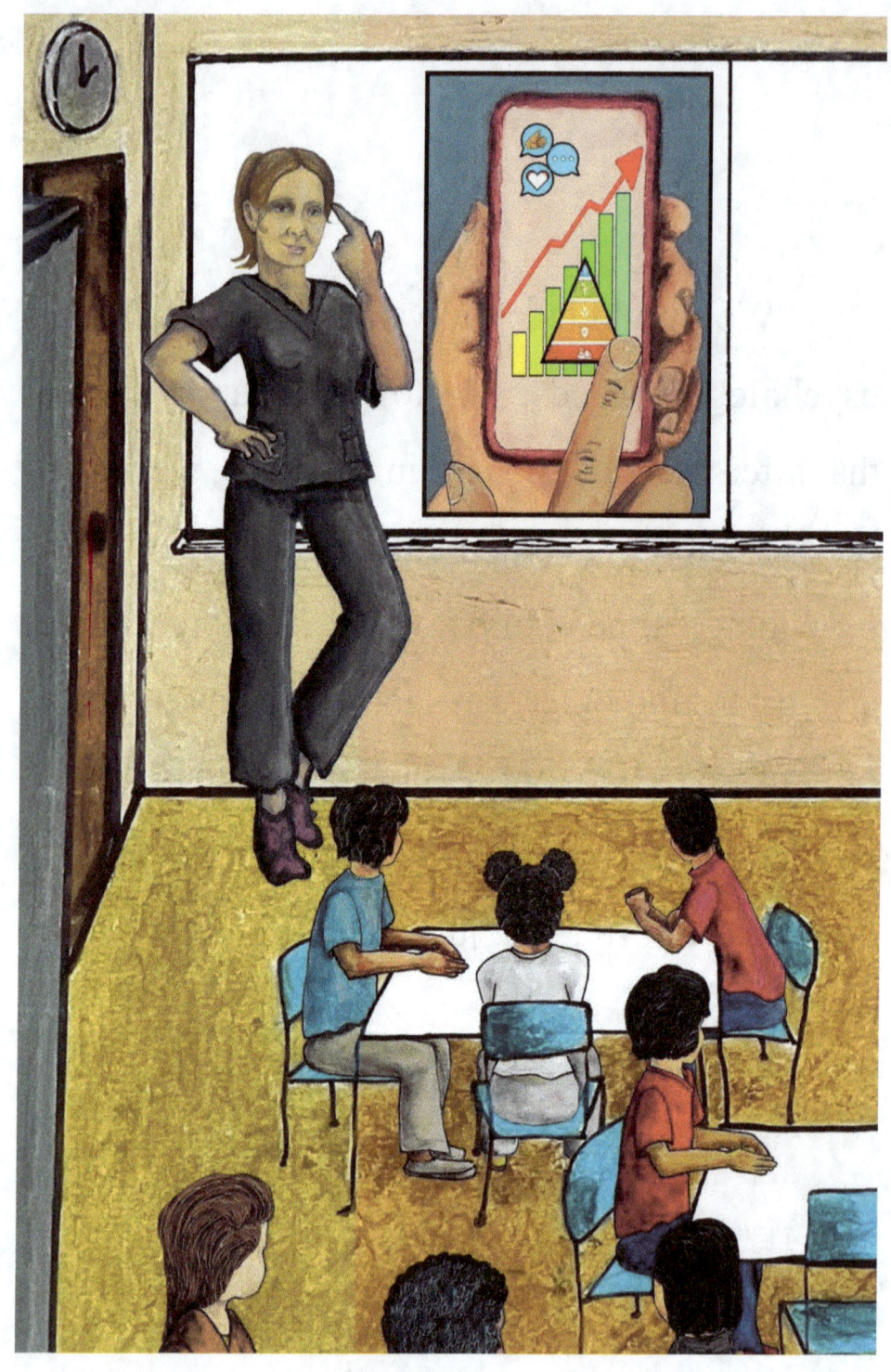

"Use social media for your different needs and motivations. Use it to make yourself a more complete person. Learn to know yourself. Become a well-rounded person that is complex, since life itself is complex."

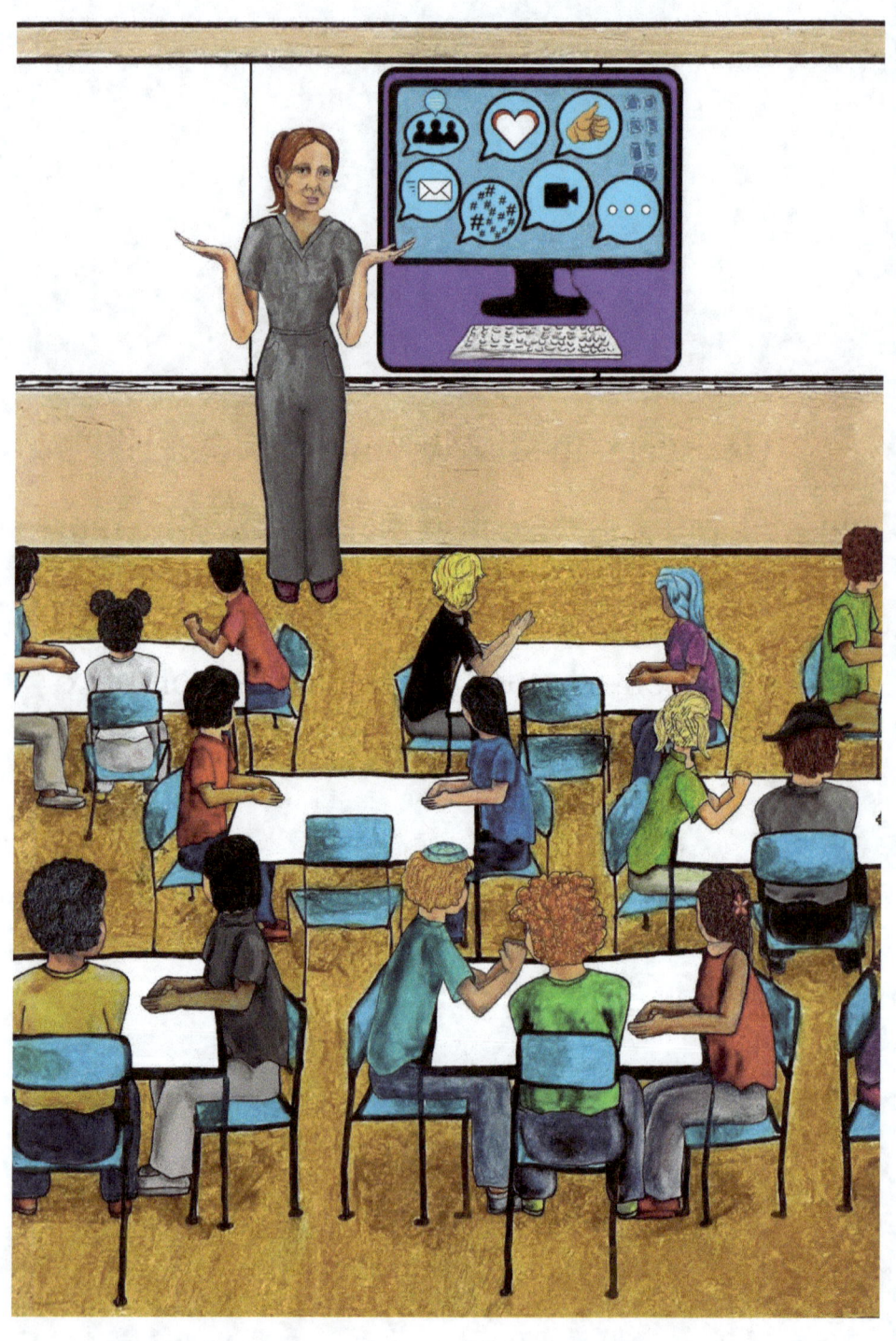

"Learn the different types of social media platforms available and use many different ones since they can have different purposes. Don't just be a user of social media, but become an integrator. Integrate these tools into your life to have a higher quality of life. Let that be one of your goals on your journey so that these tools help you instead of your using a tool just because you think you're supposed to use a social media platform."

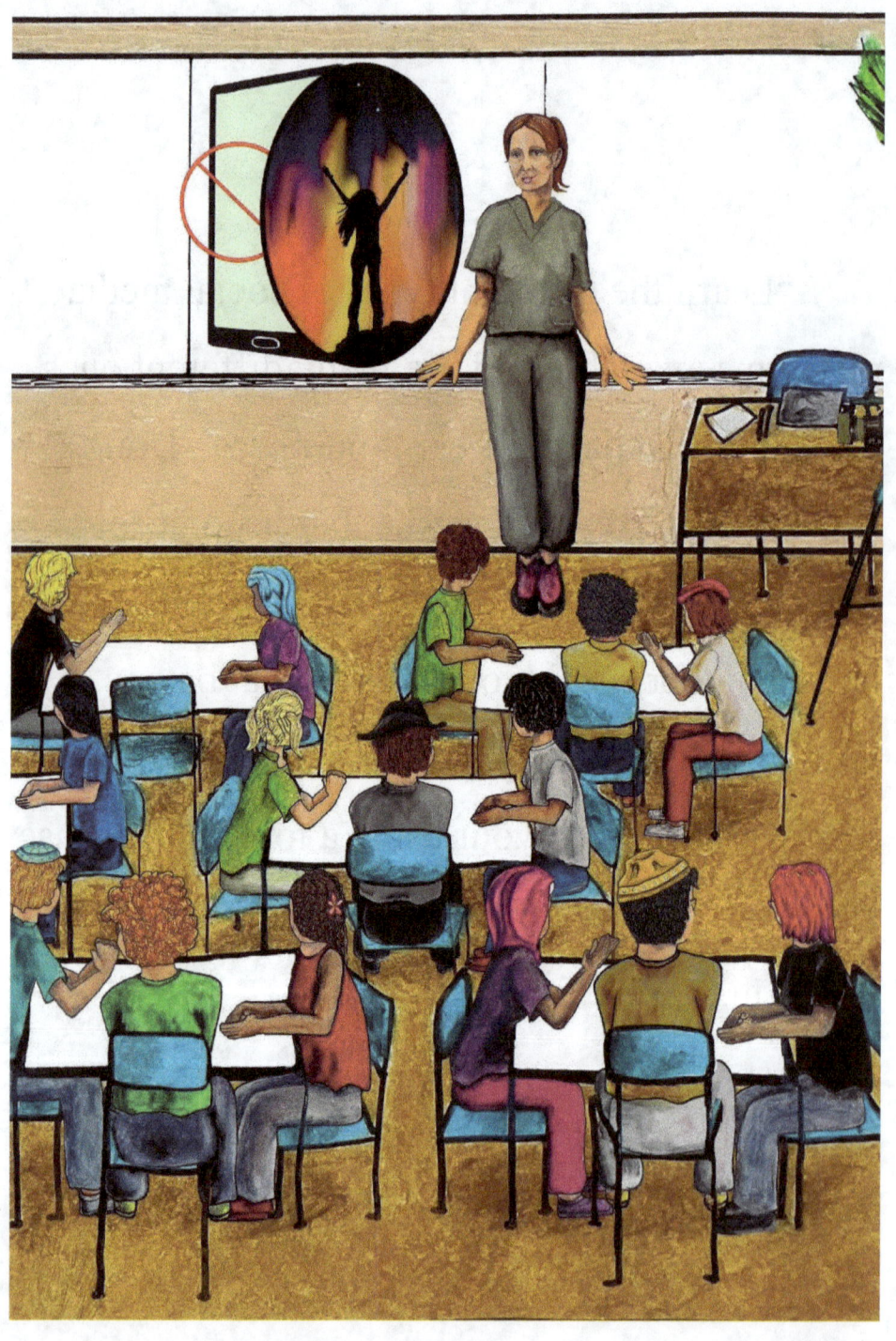

"Work on your offline well-being every day. The digital world is important, but the foundation of our lives is our physical world. Don't seek to escape life, but seek to improve life so that it is better for the next generation."

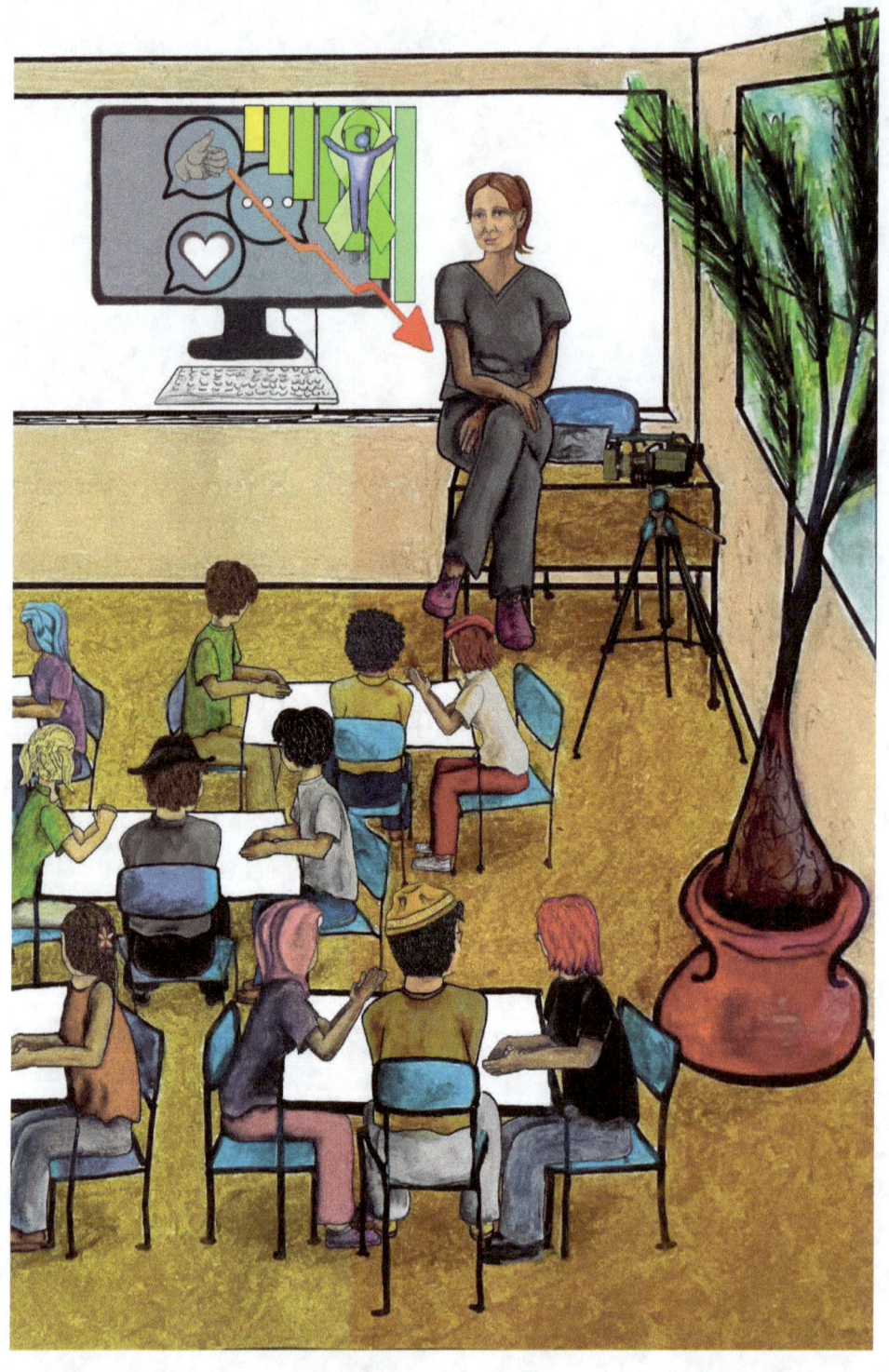

"Be cautious about using social media for something that is lacking in your life. Address problems head-on. Face your fears. Develop solutions. Implement plans. Evaluate outcomes. Adjust plans to achieve the best outcome in your life. Adapt. Evolve. Grow. Move forward in all areas of your life."

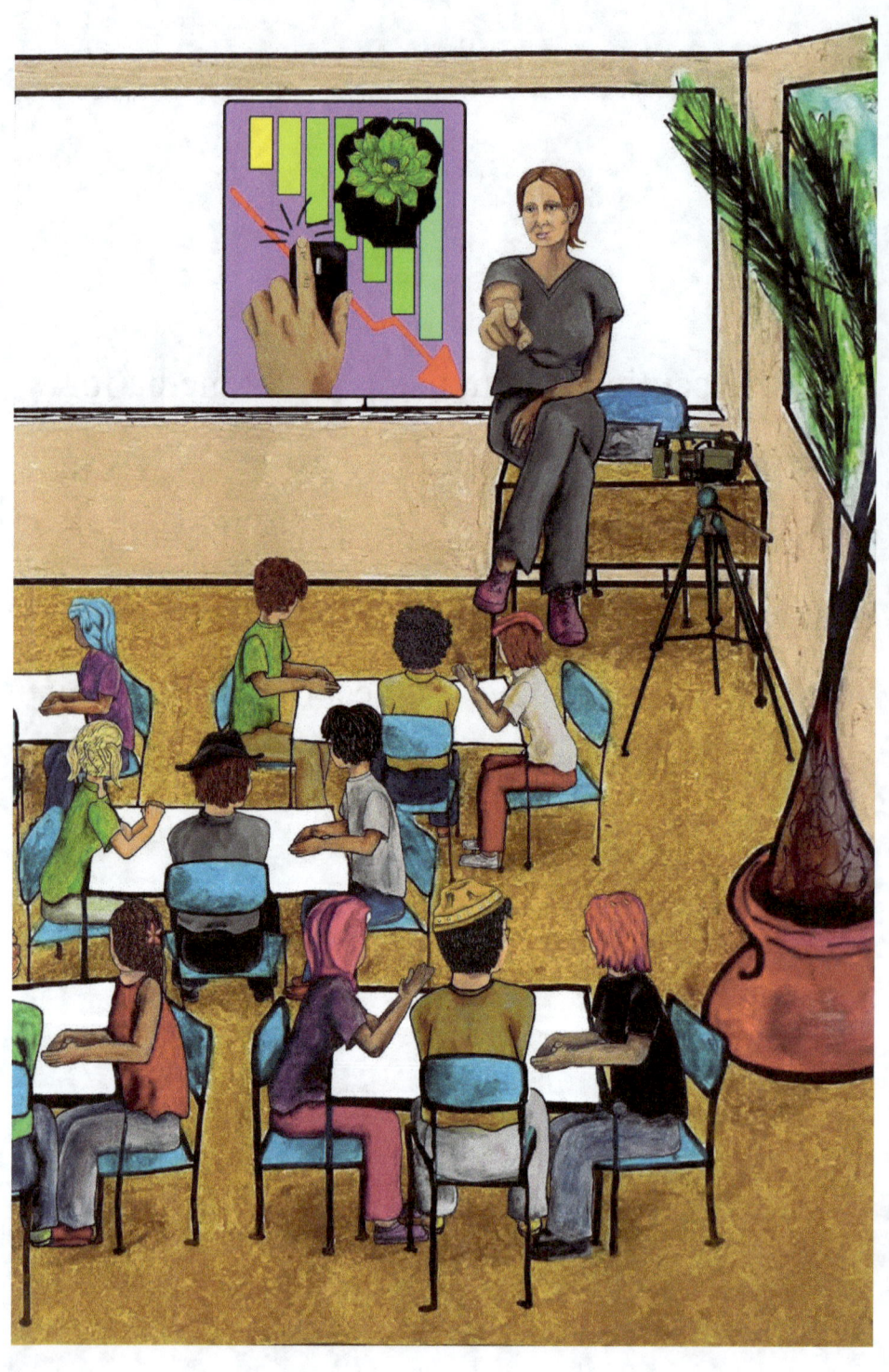

"Some research shows social media can decrease well-being if it is passive like just scrolling and watching short videos. Well-being can be enhanced if you are more active in your social media like interacting with comments."

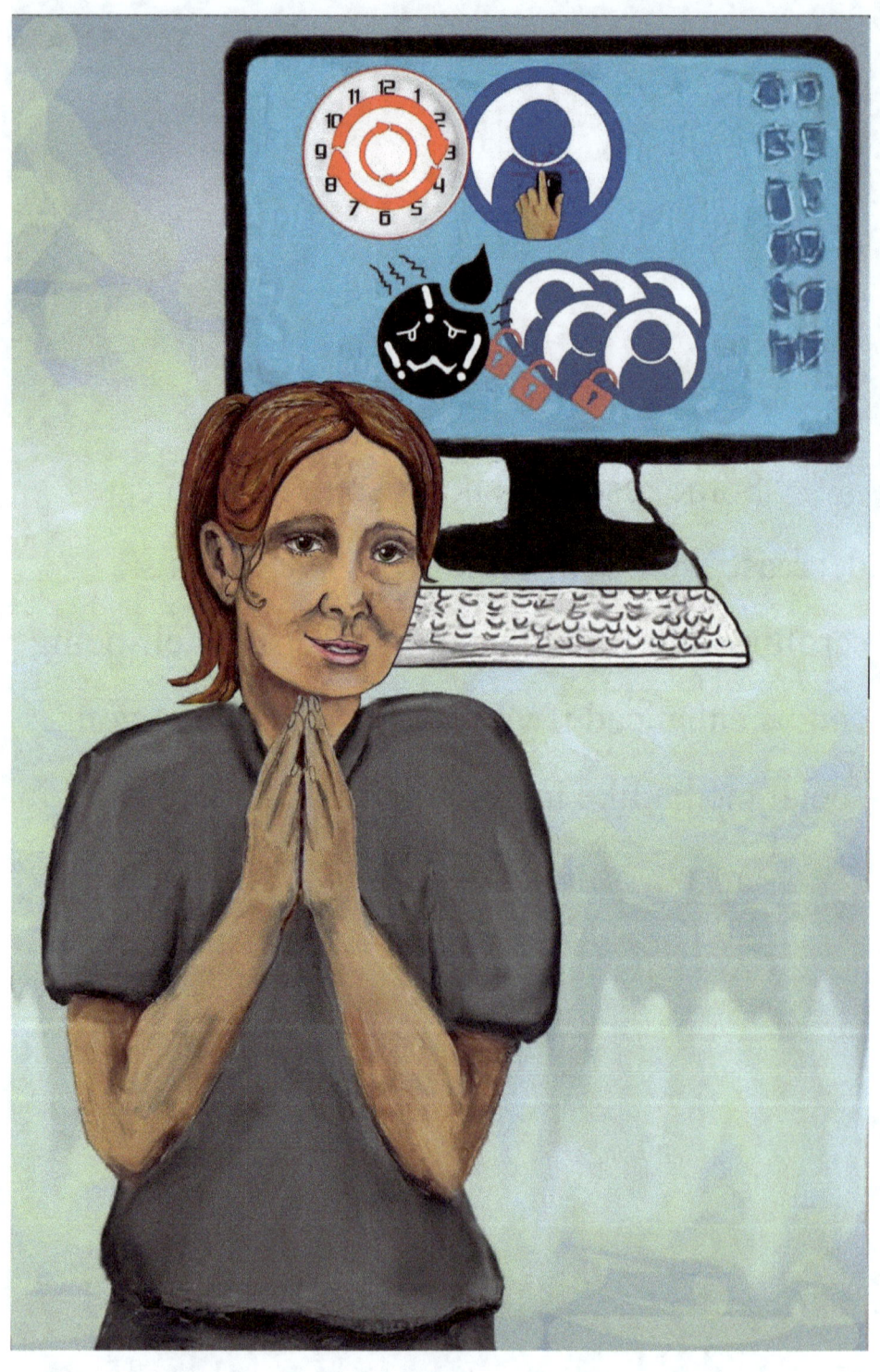

"Routine use may not be a problem, but it can cause some problems if you are checking apps excessively because you fear missing out or are disappointed if your friends are not logged in."

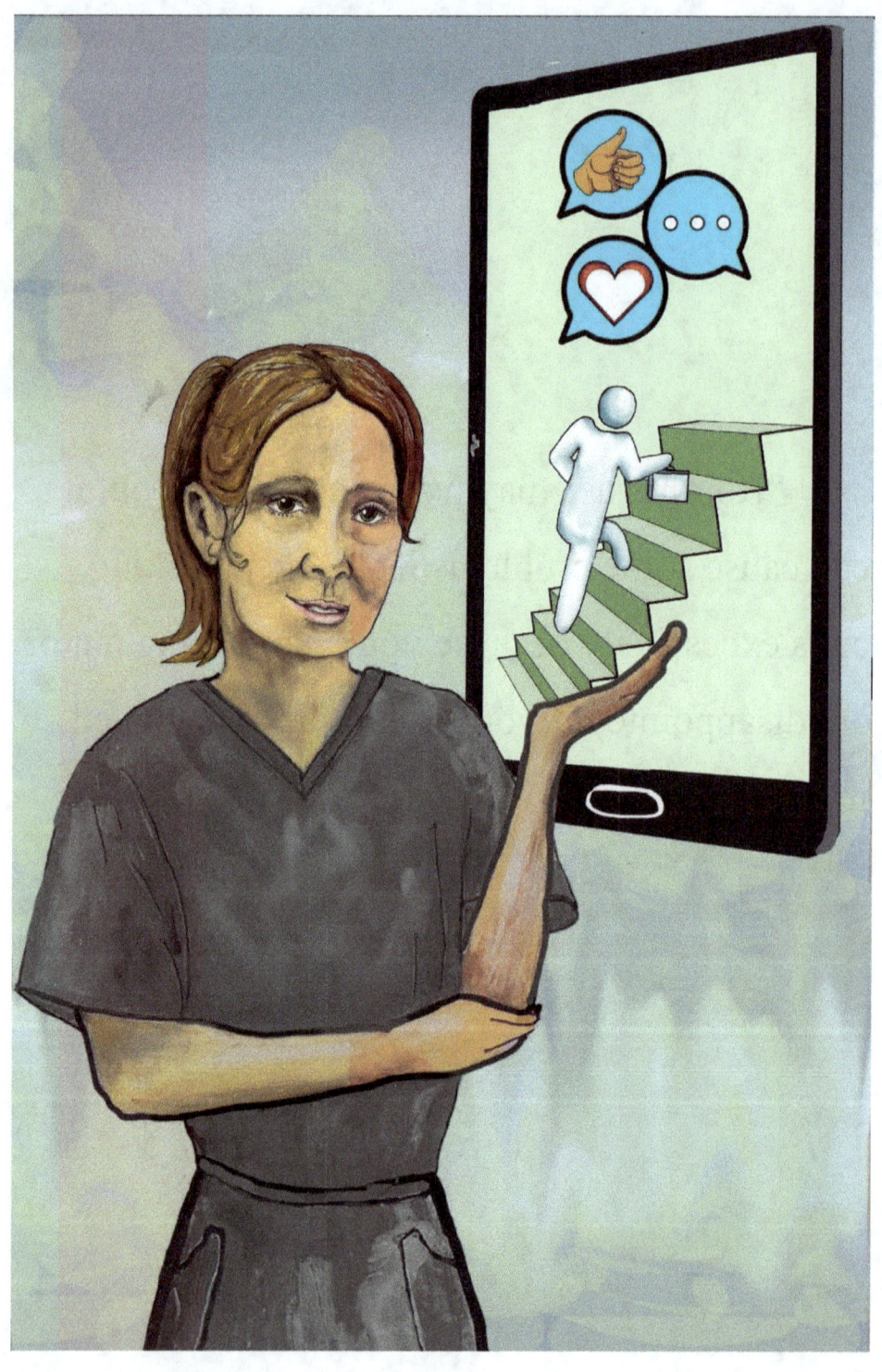

"Once you start a career, use social media to better your work life. Use social media to get tips on how to be a better co-worker as well as how to work more efficiently so you can be identified for promotion."

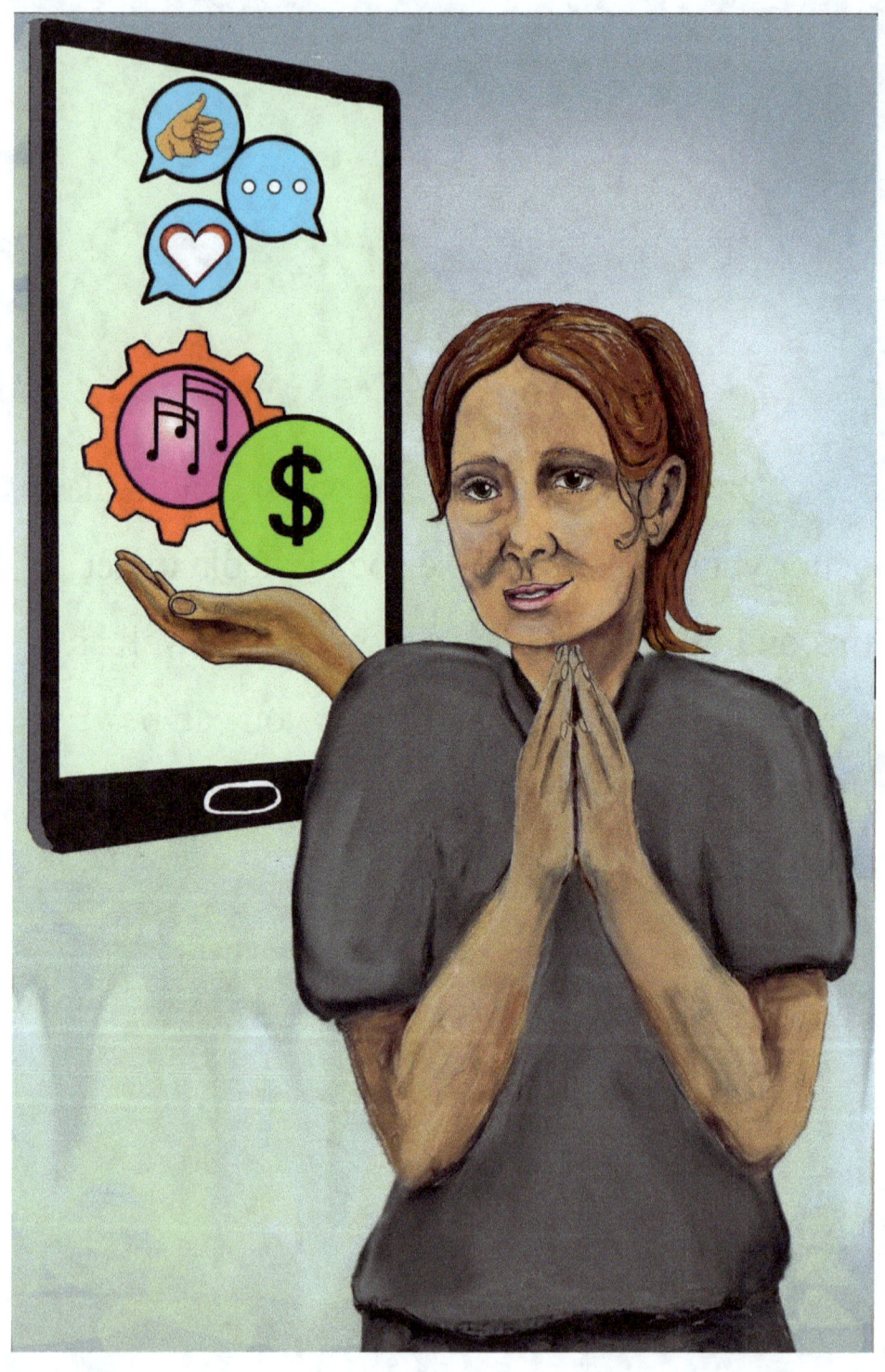

"You could use social media to do a side gig and earn some extra money, so that you can buy the things you need or take a nice vacation that you otherwise may not have been able to."

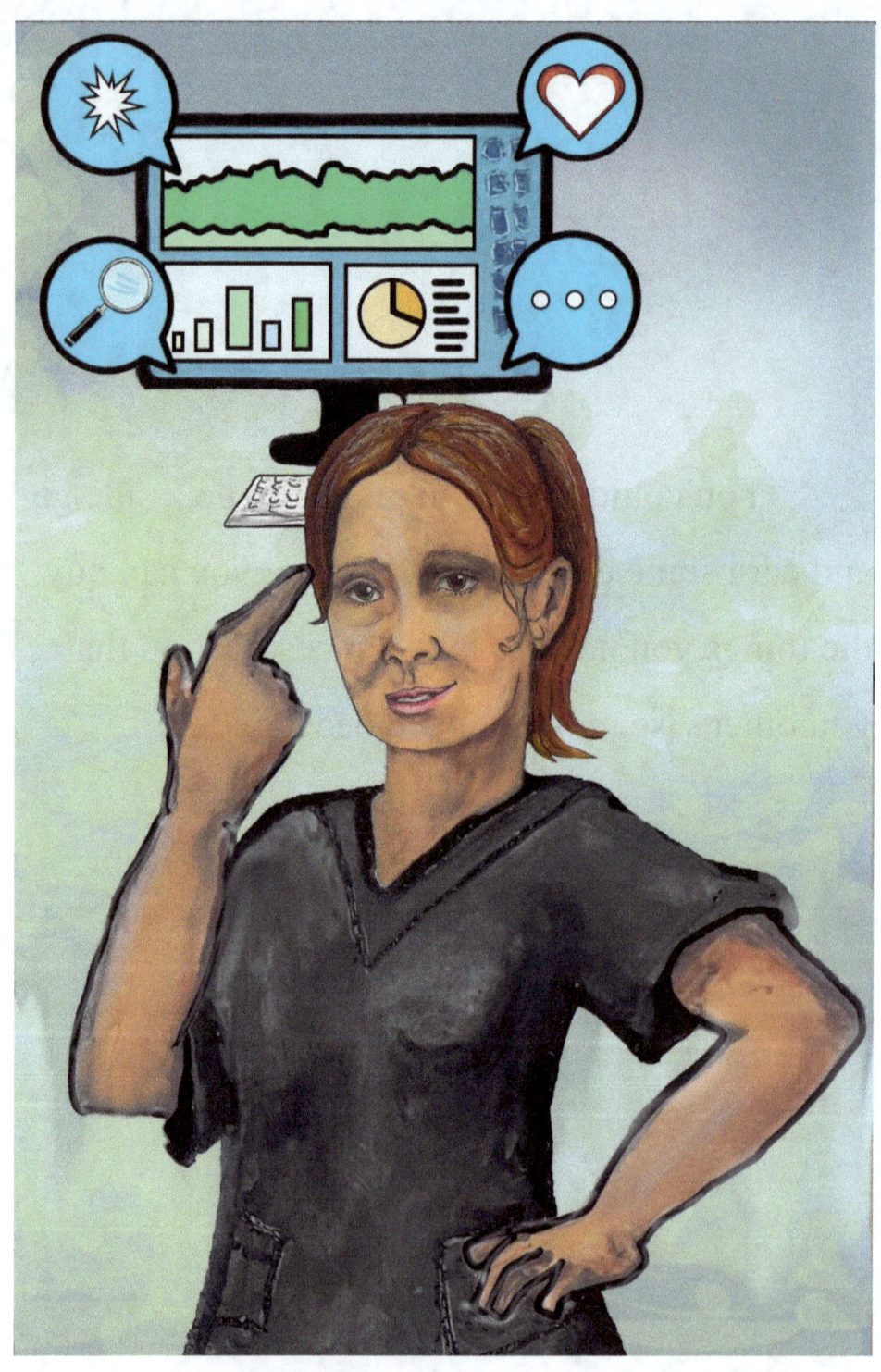

"Developing effortful control is important for social media moderation. This type of control is your ability to regulate your emotions and behaviors. Developing effortful control can help you moderate your social media use as well as help you use social media for constructive purposes. It involves developing longer attention spans, increasing your memory, and stopping impulsive behaviors so that you accomplish goals. Seek to find errors in your thinking and behaviors, and plan ahead."

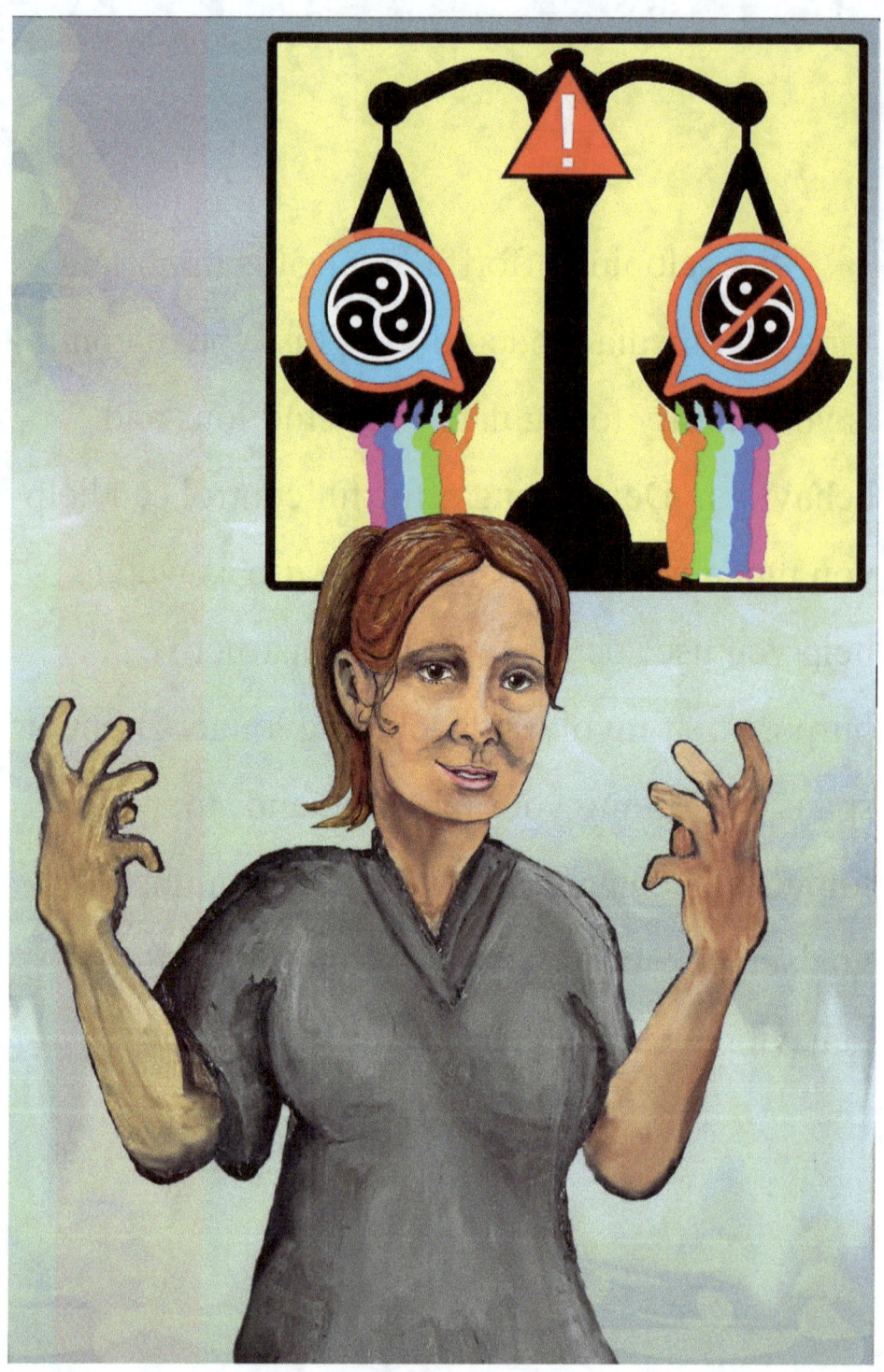

"Effortful control is defined as the ability to withhold a dominant response in order to perform a nondominant response. This allows a person to detect errors, to engage in planning, and to involve executive attention. This allows children to come to regulate their more reactive and impulsive tendencies."

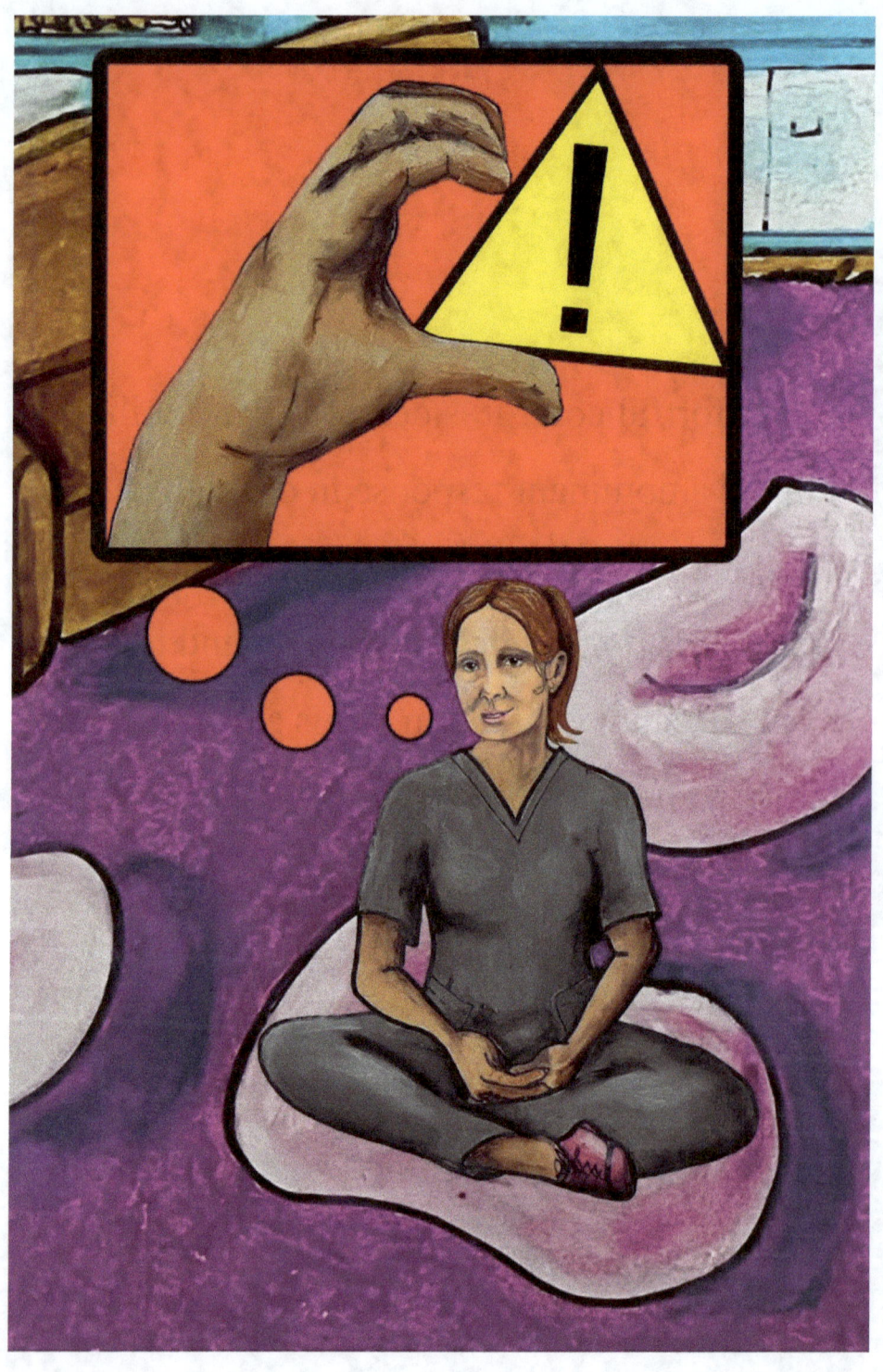

"Attentional regulation involves the development of the skills of selective attention, focus, attention switching, and multitasking. Skills are things you must do many times to get good at them. If you think that you're not good at multitasking, you may be correct, so you need to practice multitasking more."

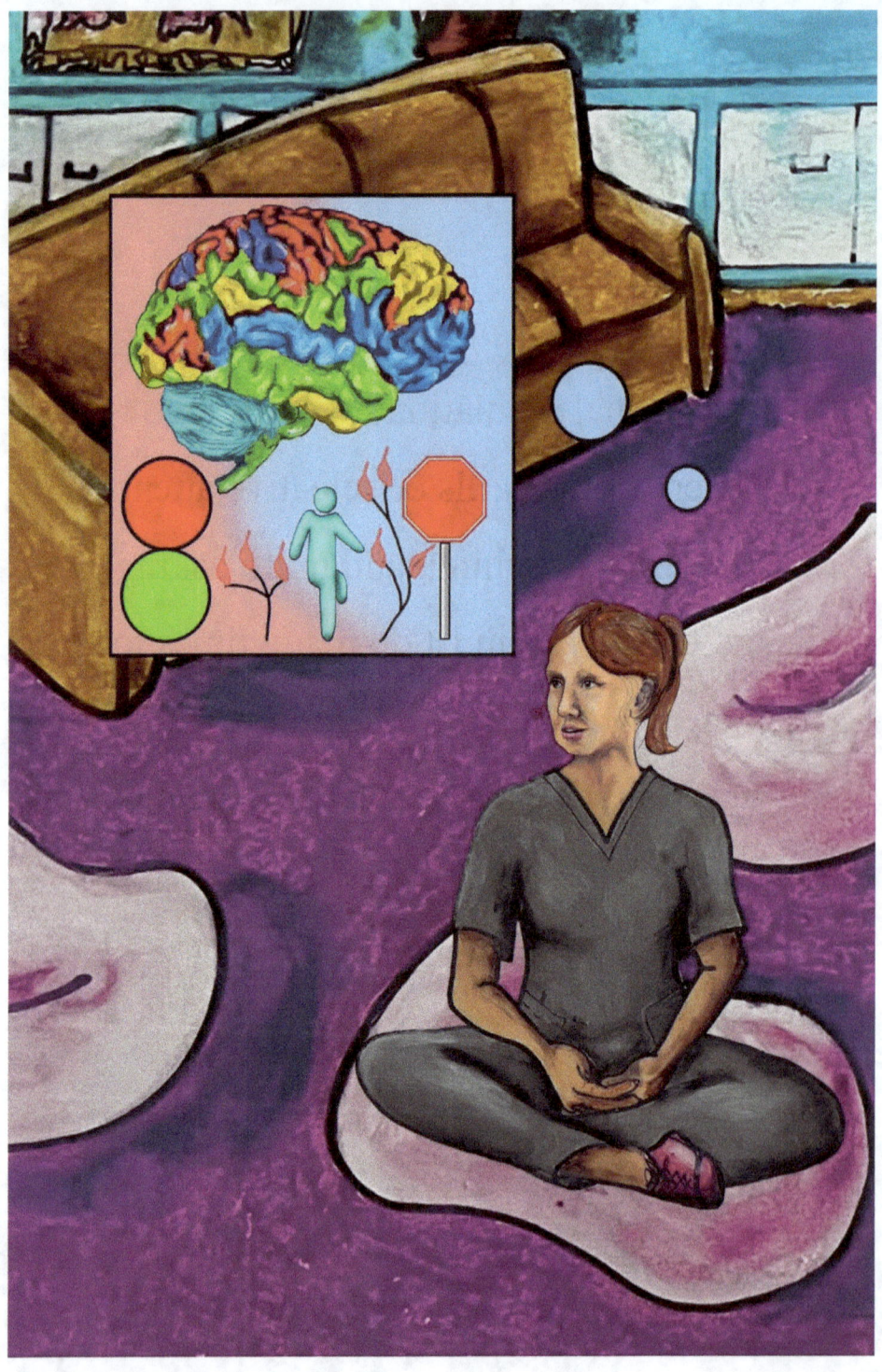

"Inhibitory control with effortful control is suppressing behaviors that are inappropriate or that will lead to poor results. If you are not good at suppressing behaviors, it is because it is a skill. Try to stop behaviors that are inappropriate in a safe place and environment so that when you are somewhere public, it may be easier to suppress the behavior that is socially inappropriate."

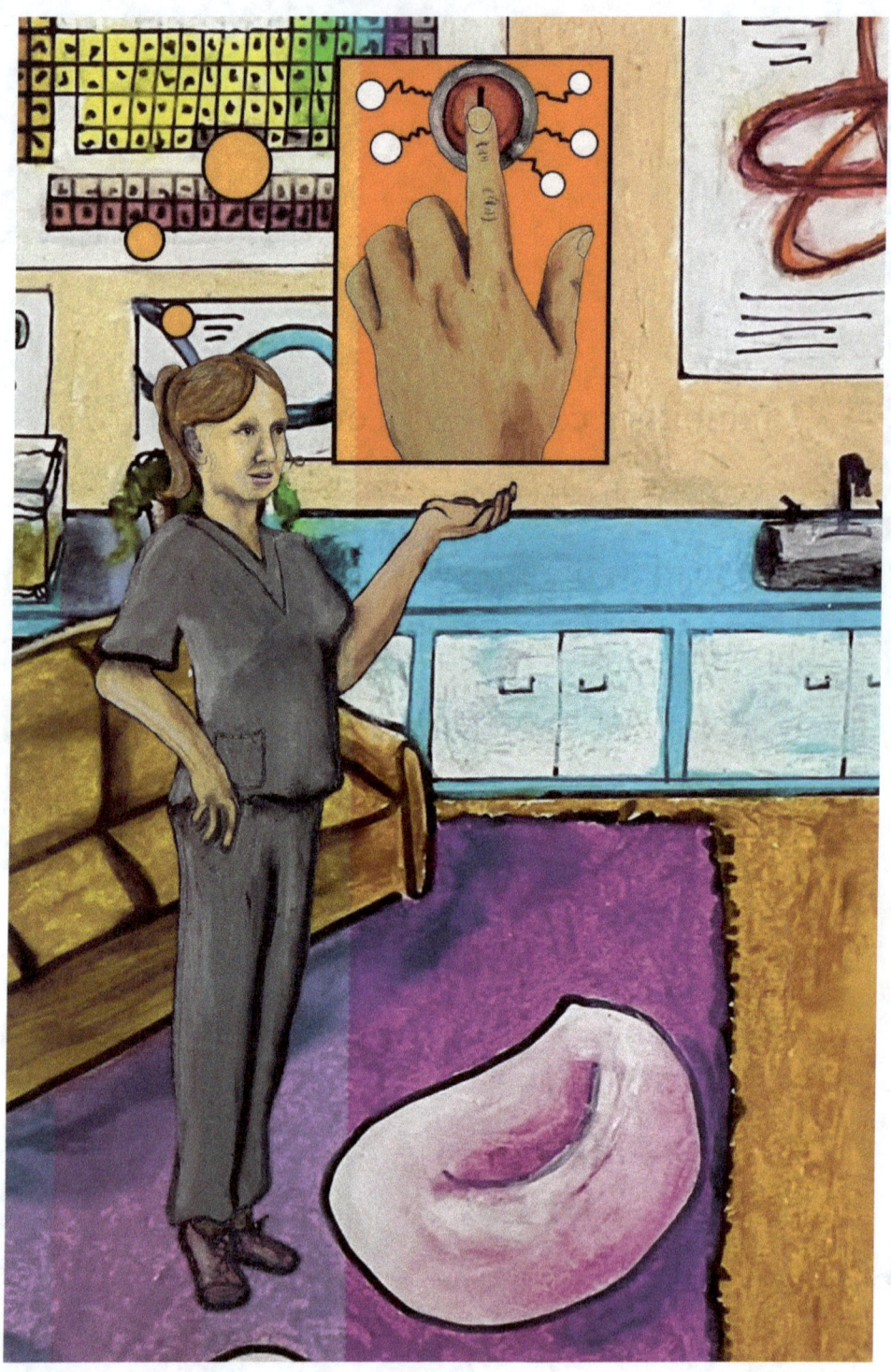

"Activational control is something involved in effortful control. This is when you activate certain behaviors so that either you get the rewards you want, or that they are behaviors that are socially appropriate for the situation. An example would be to say comforting things to someone being bullied so that they feel supported and not alone."

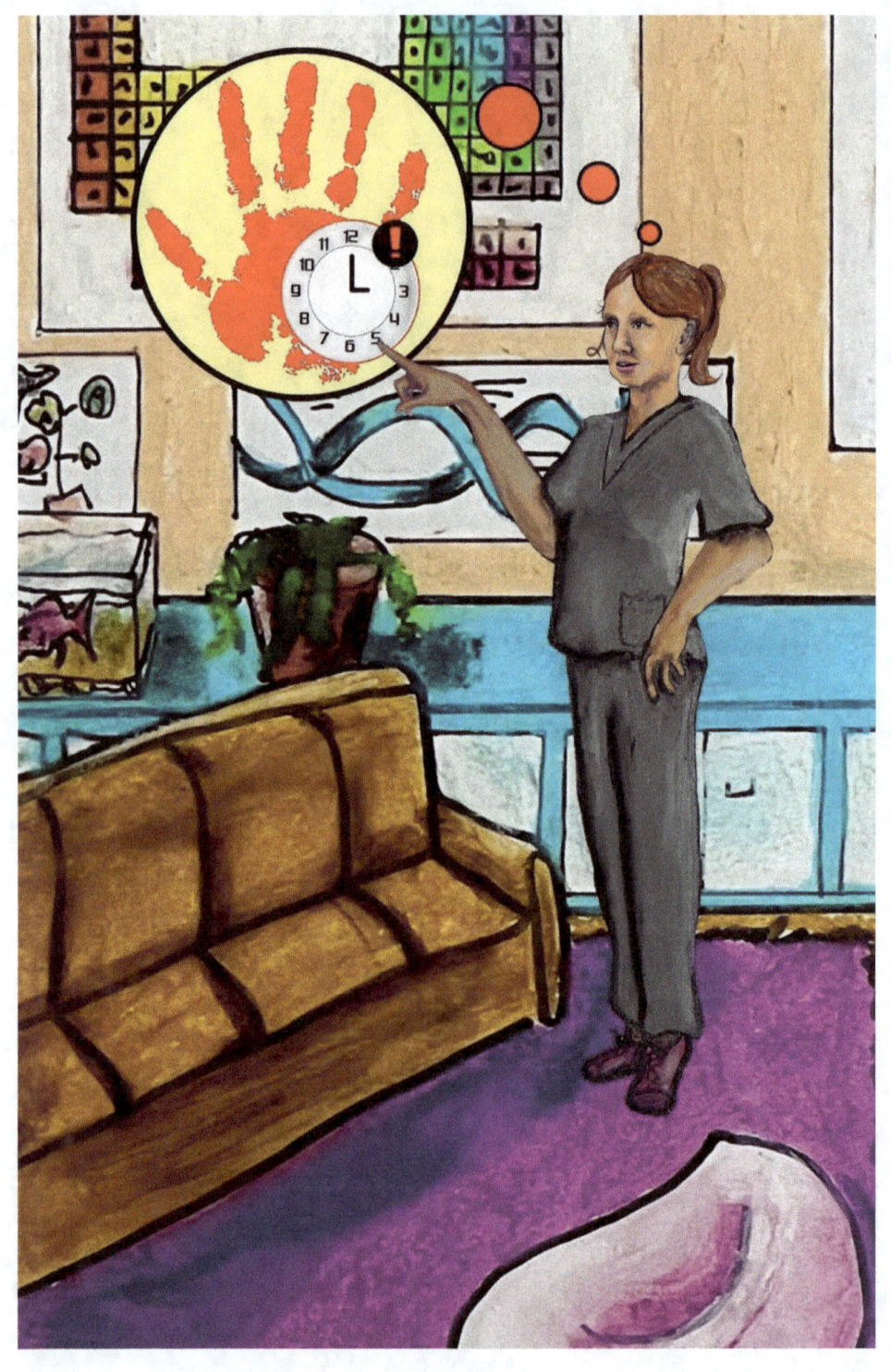

"Delay is an effortful control skill. It is developing the ability to delay gratification such as waiting for candy."

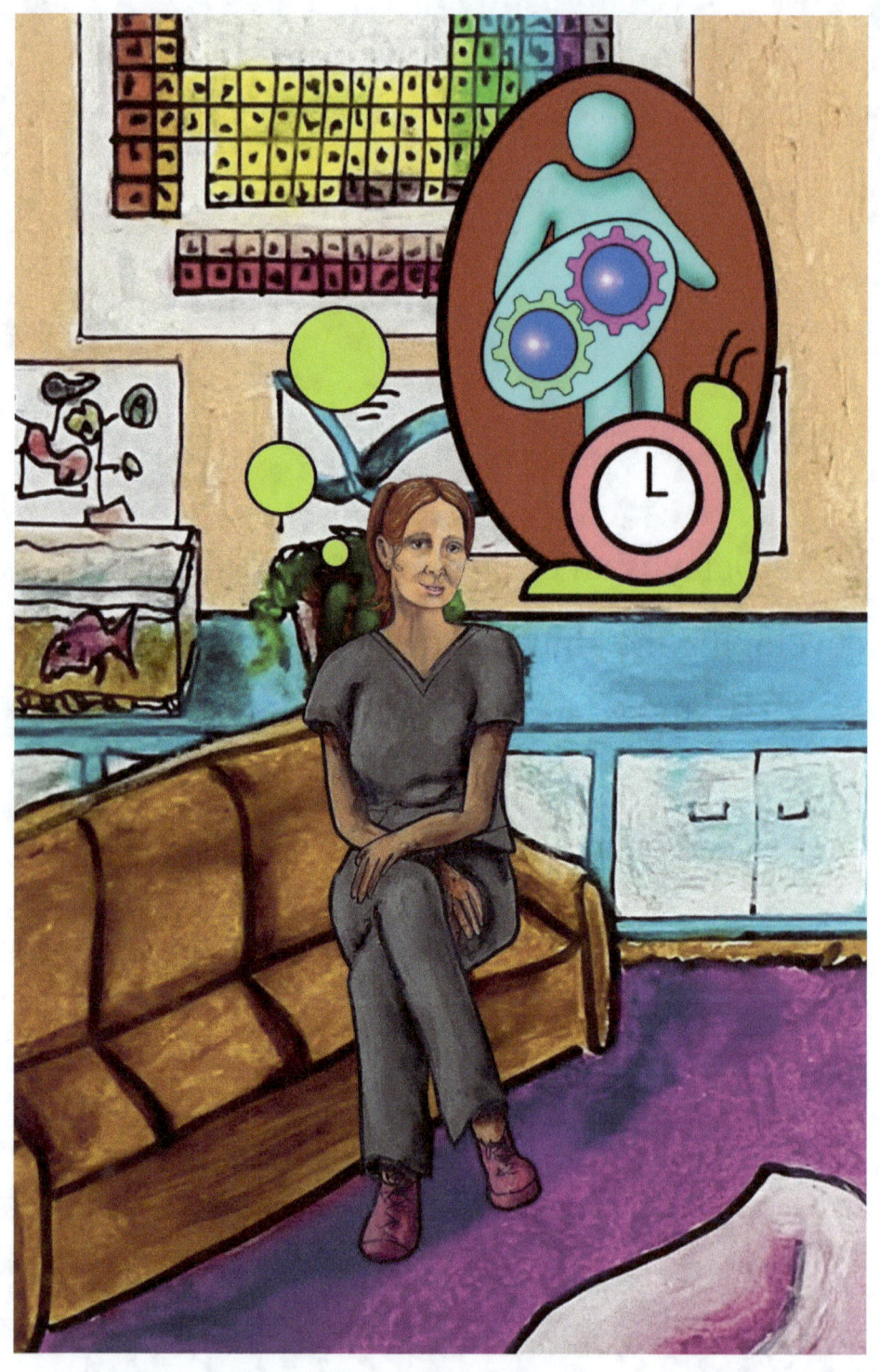

"Another skill is slowing down motor movement. An example of this would be to slowly draw a line instead of scribbling."

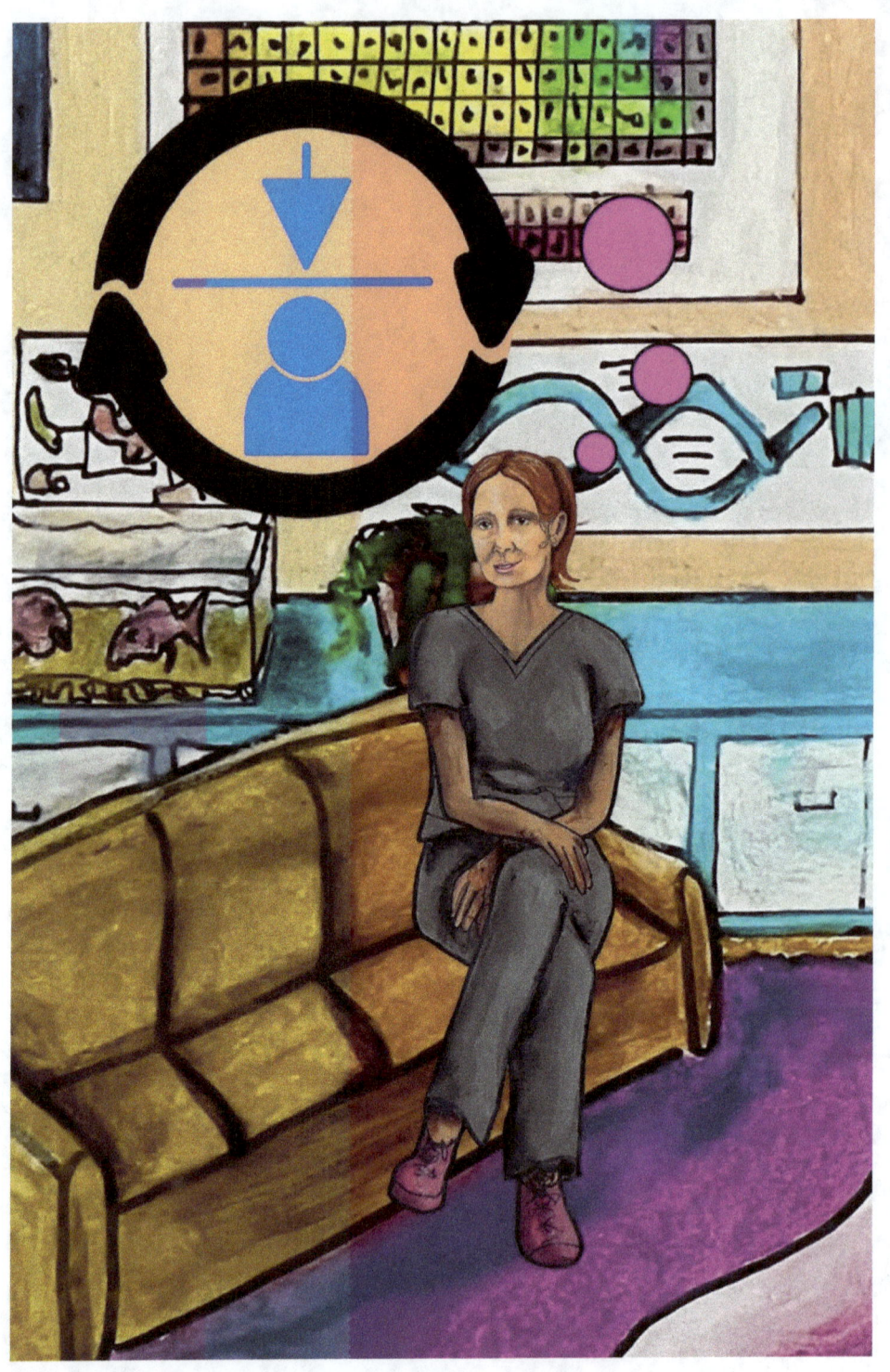

"A third skill for effortful control is suppressing and initiating responses to changing signals. An example would be playing the childhood game of Simon Says. Learning to change your behavior with a new signal is important."

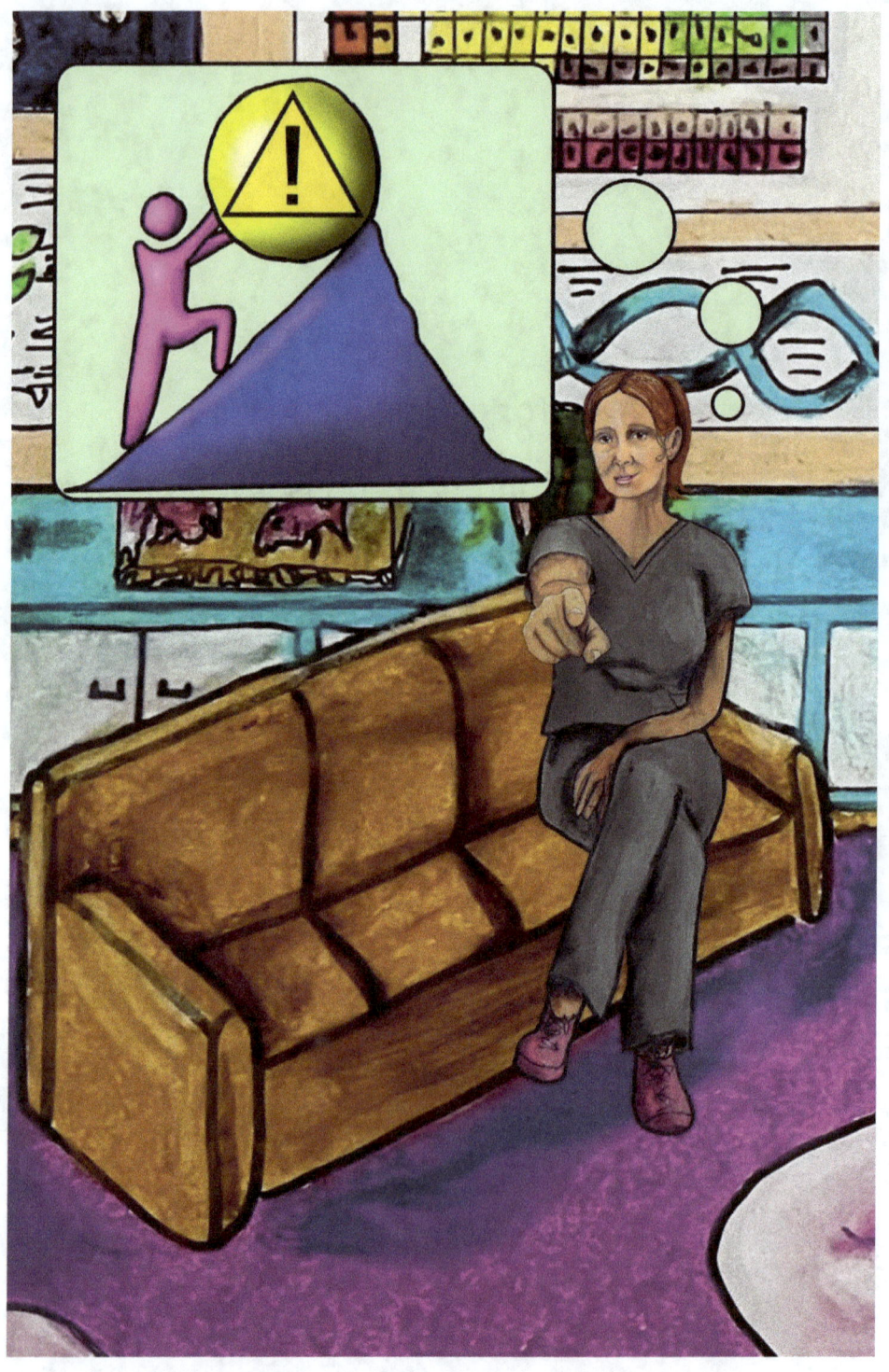

"Effortful attention is another important skill. An example would be finding small shapes hidden within a larger shape."

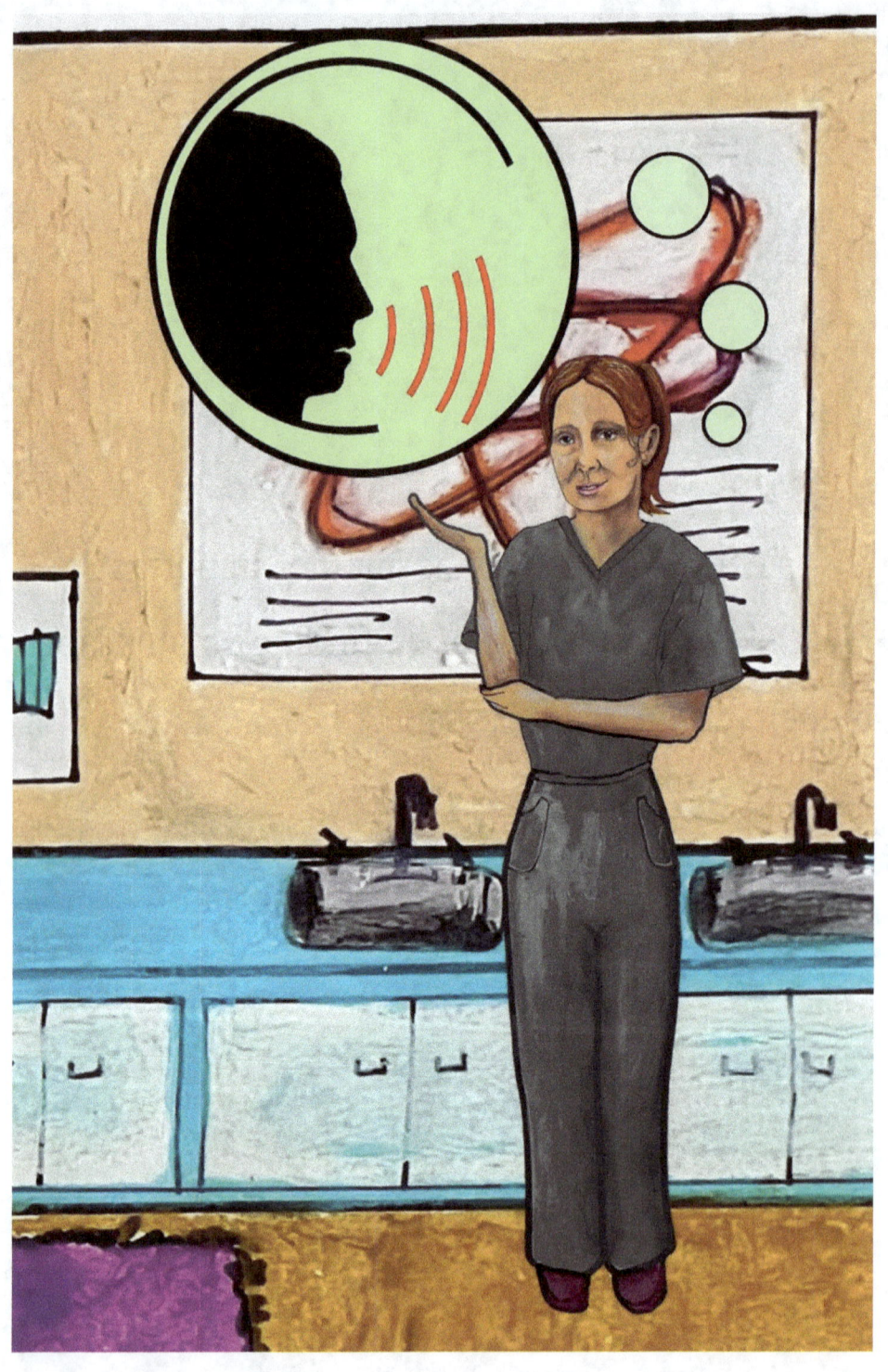

"A fifth skill is voice control. As the name implies, this is where you change the volume of your voice so that it is appropriate to the situation."

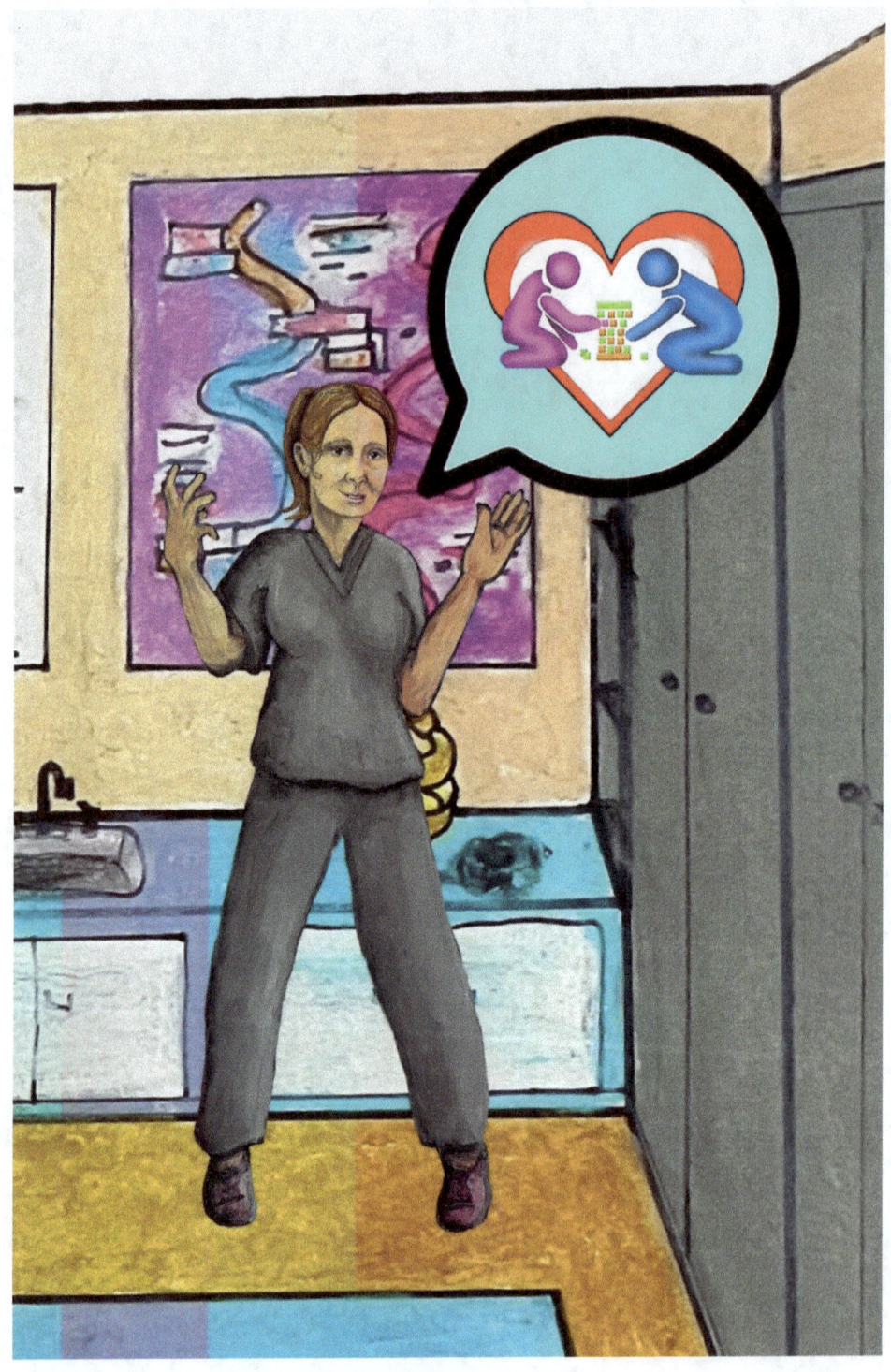

"An example of effortful control is sharing toys. By sharing something enjoyable with another person, the person not only develops social skills to interact others but also develops empathy toward others. Waiting your turn is another example of using effortful control. Waiting in line patiently is important."

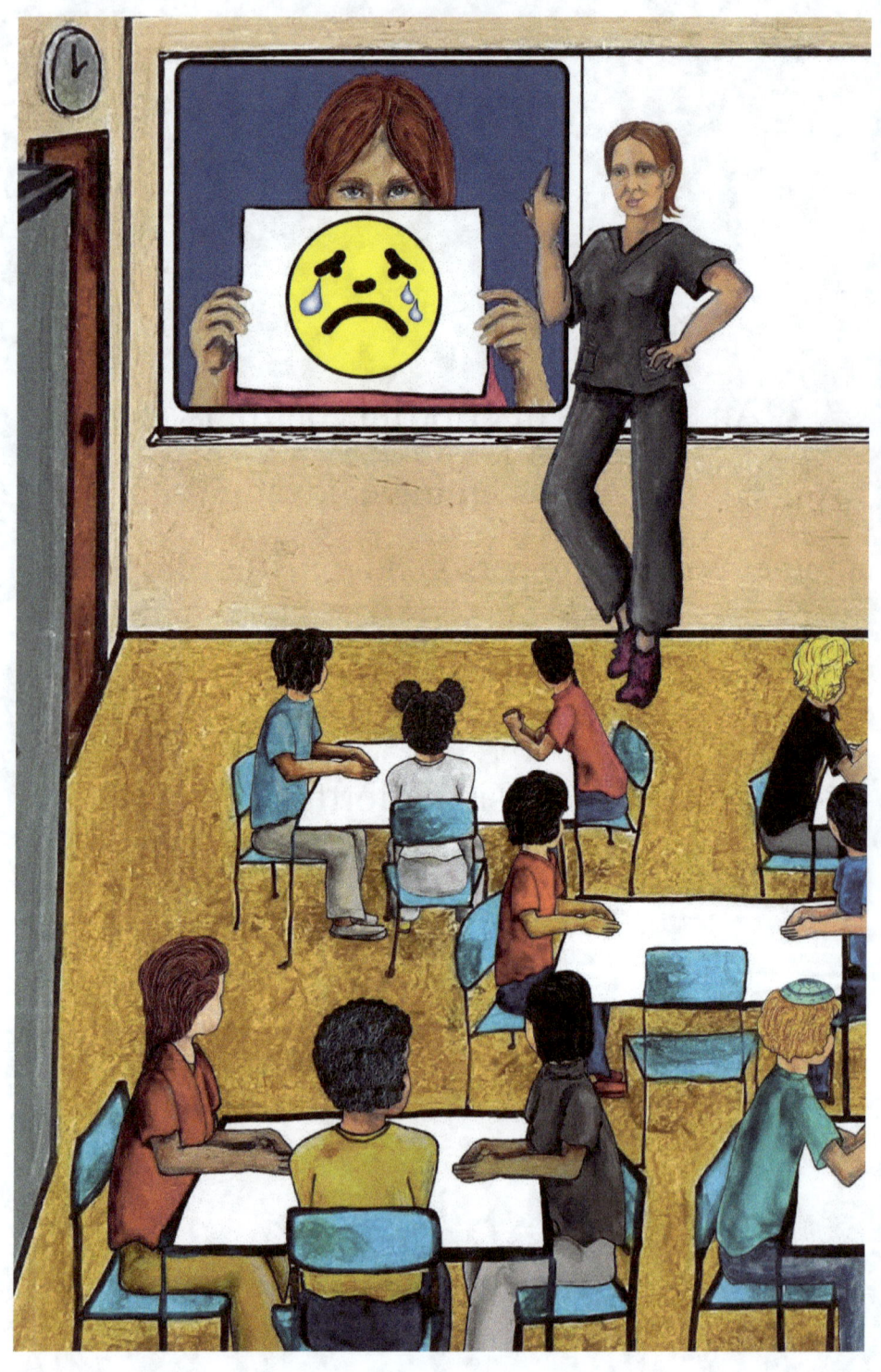

"Another example is handling disappointment well. When you get disappointed, try to not let your negative emotions control your behavior. Avoid a meltdown. Accept the situation as peacefully as possible. This helps a person become more resilient and able person to handle the ups and downs of life."

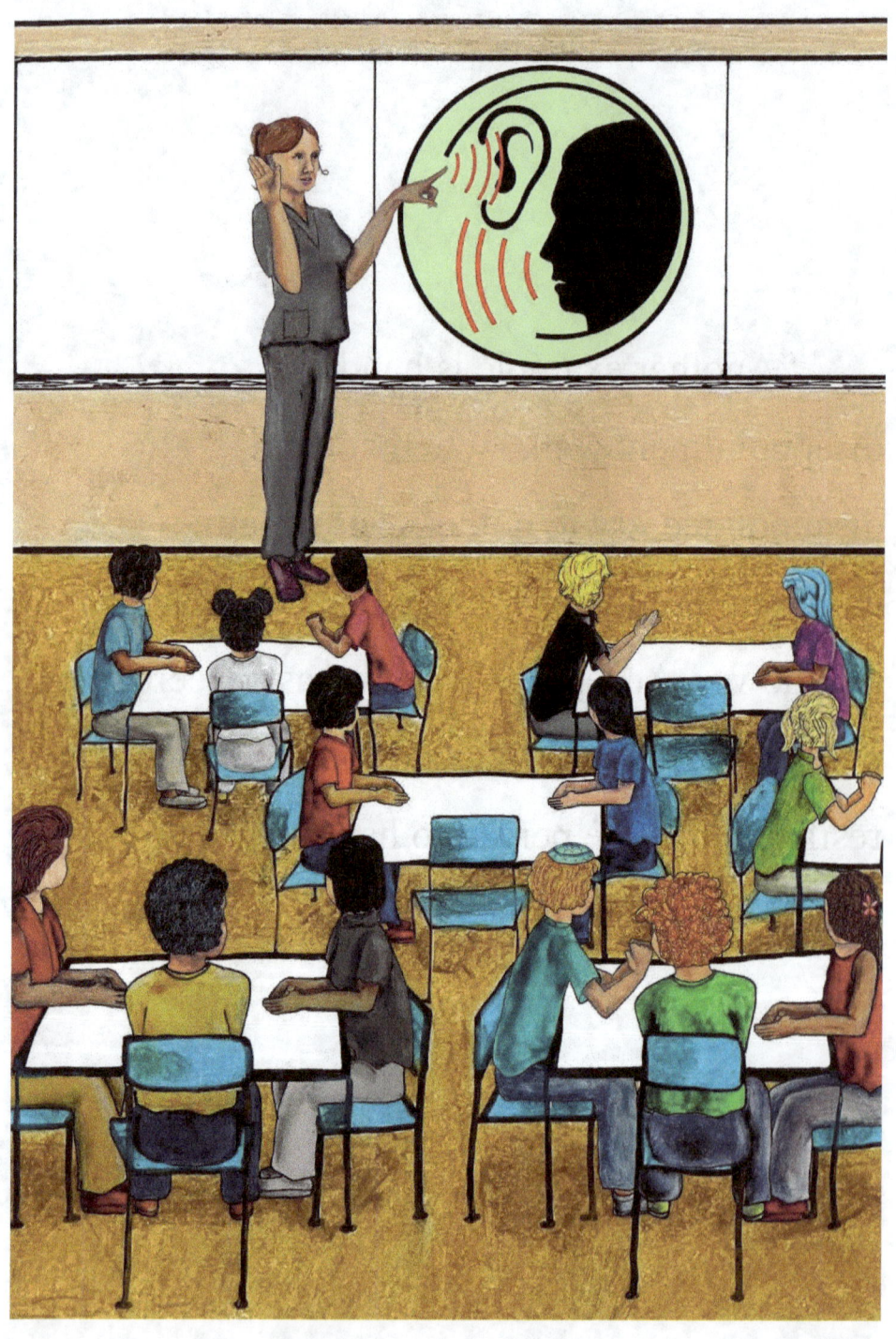

"Listening in class or during a group instruction is another example of effortful control. Avoid talking to friends while the instructor is talking. Give your attention to the teacher. Try to interact with educational material."

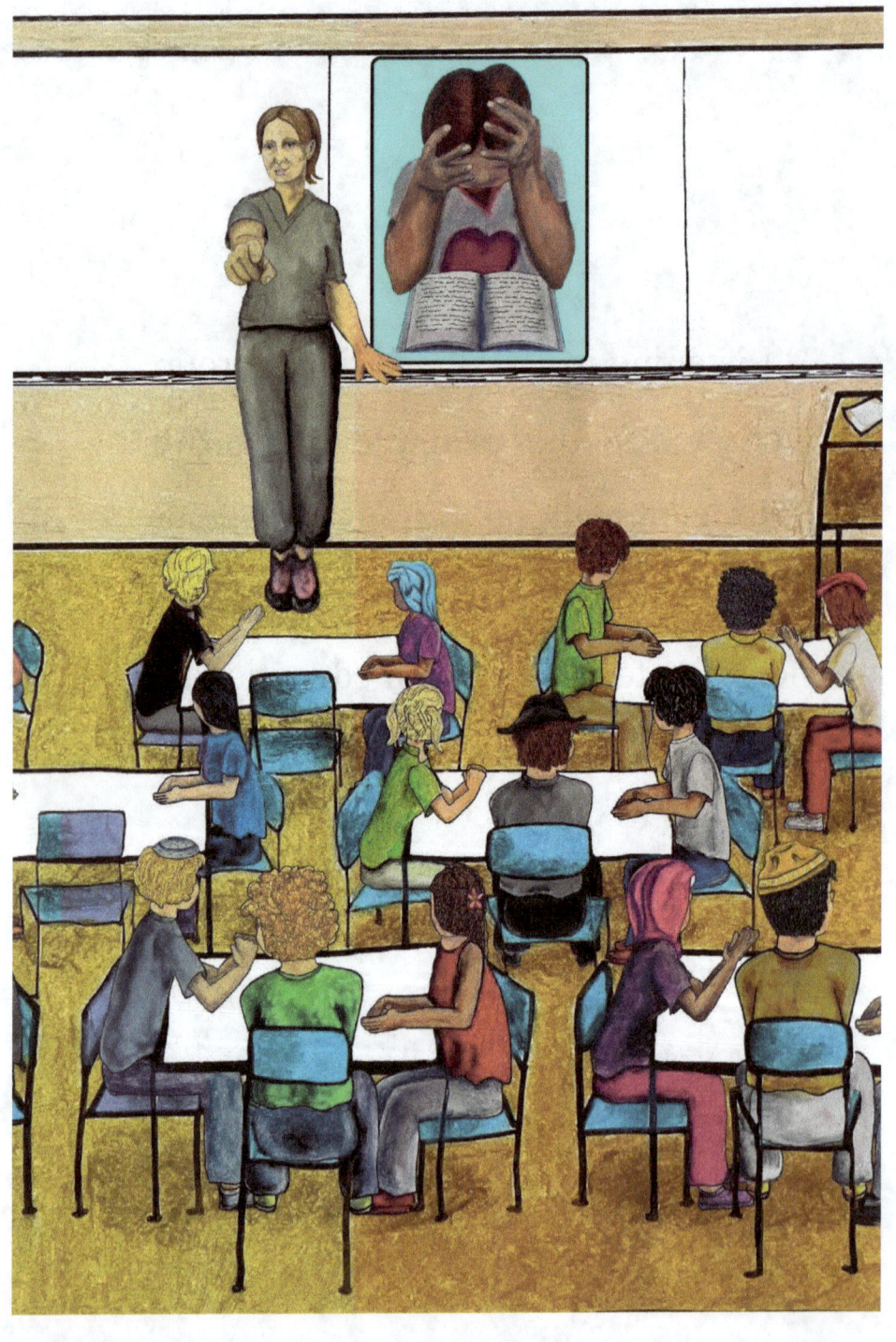

"A fifth example of effortful control is completing homework. Put your distractions to the side and focus on your task. Having a strong work ethic is very important in life. Studying for an exam is another example. You might need to find a quiet place to study. You may have to choose to study over doing something entertaining such as using social media. Prioritizing is a skill that all humans must learn."

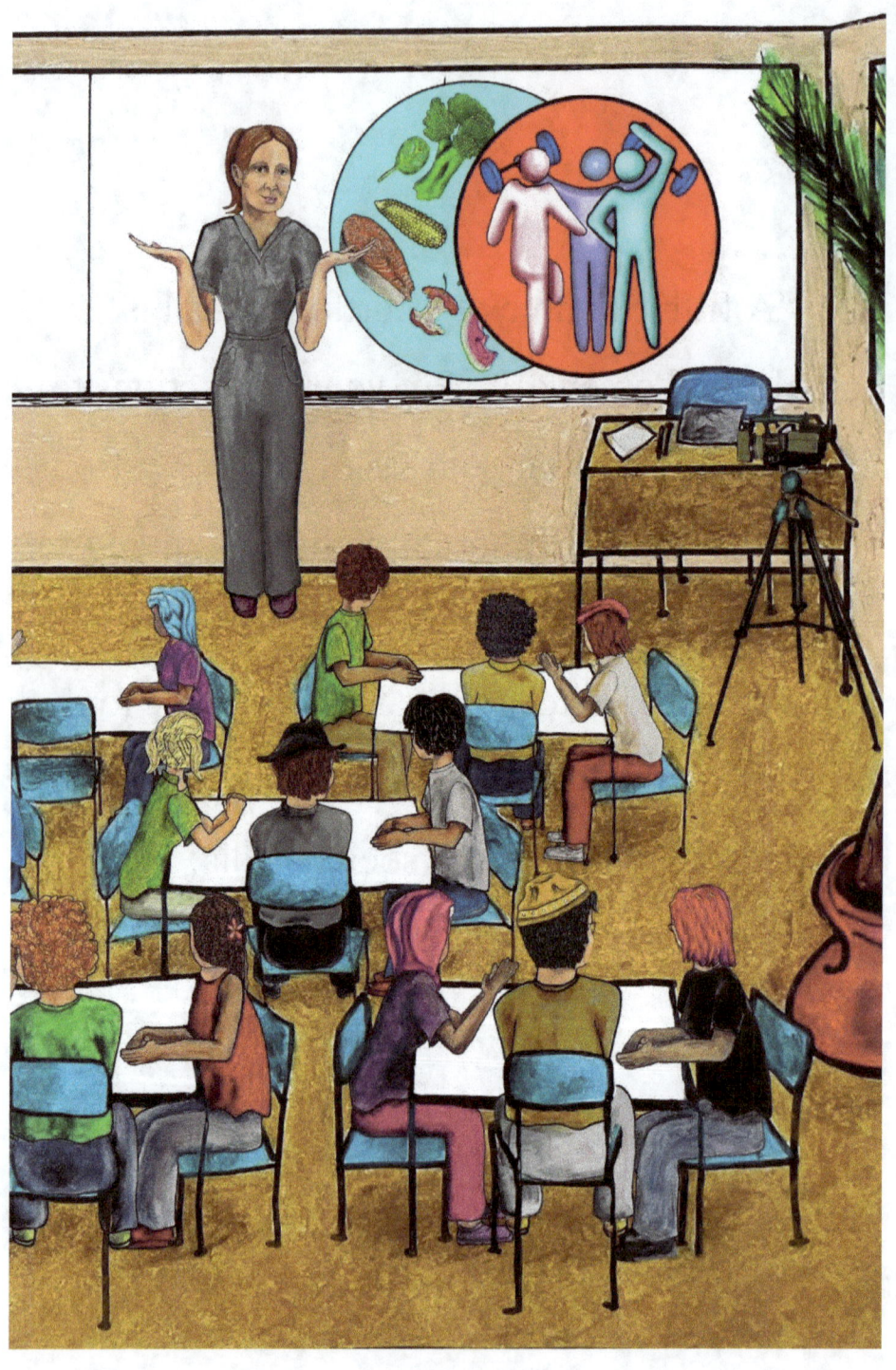

"Keeping a healthy diet and exercising are other examples of effortful control. You may need to stop yourself from eating too many sugary foods. You may need to stop yourself from overeating. You may need to exercise on days that you just don't feel like it. Having a diet and exercise partner really helps with developing these habits."

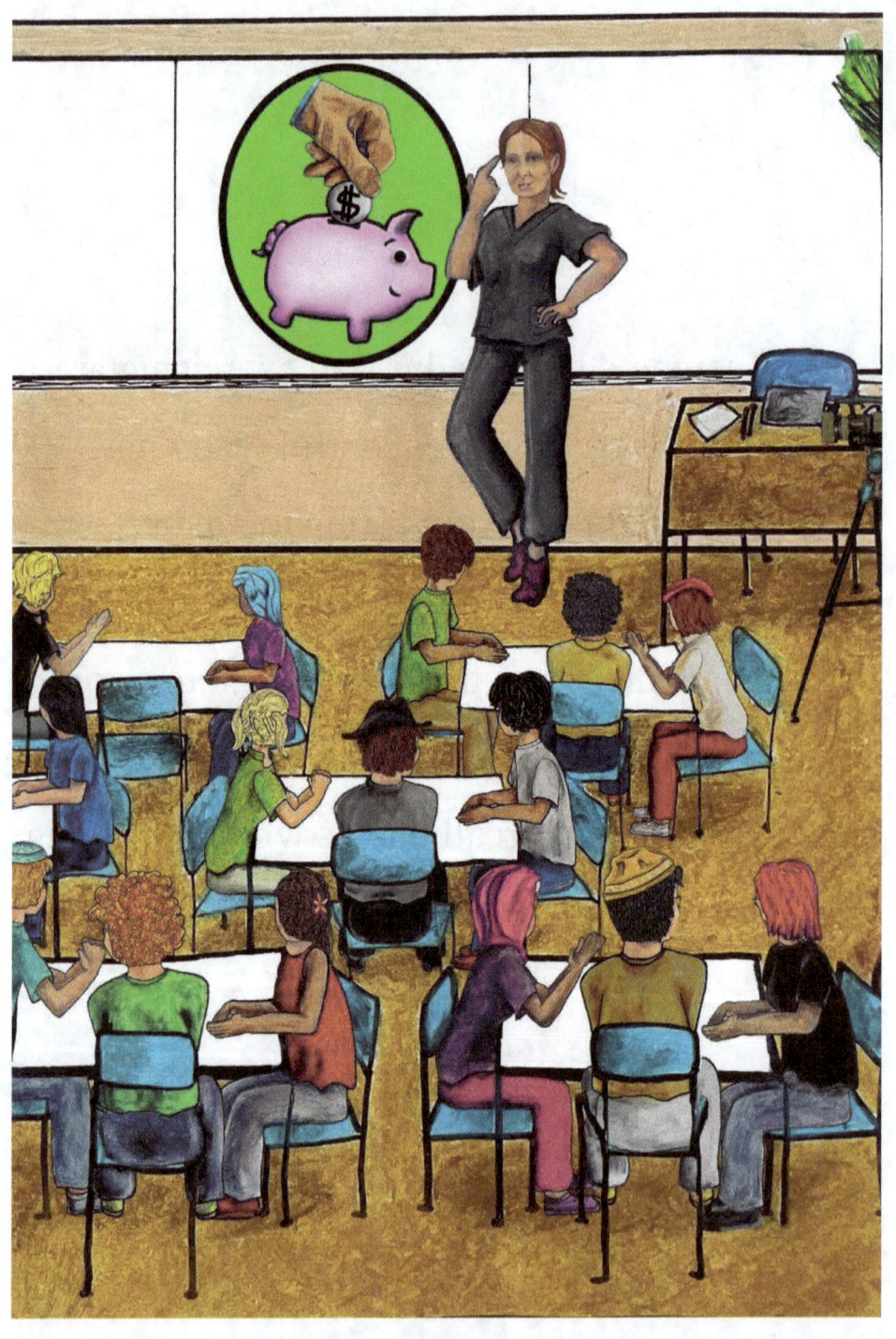

"Saving money is another example. This requires a person to not spend impulsively. Try to develop a budget and then stick to it. Use receipts and track your expenses at the end of each week to make sure you are actually keeping your budget."

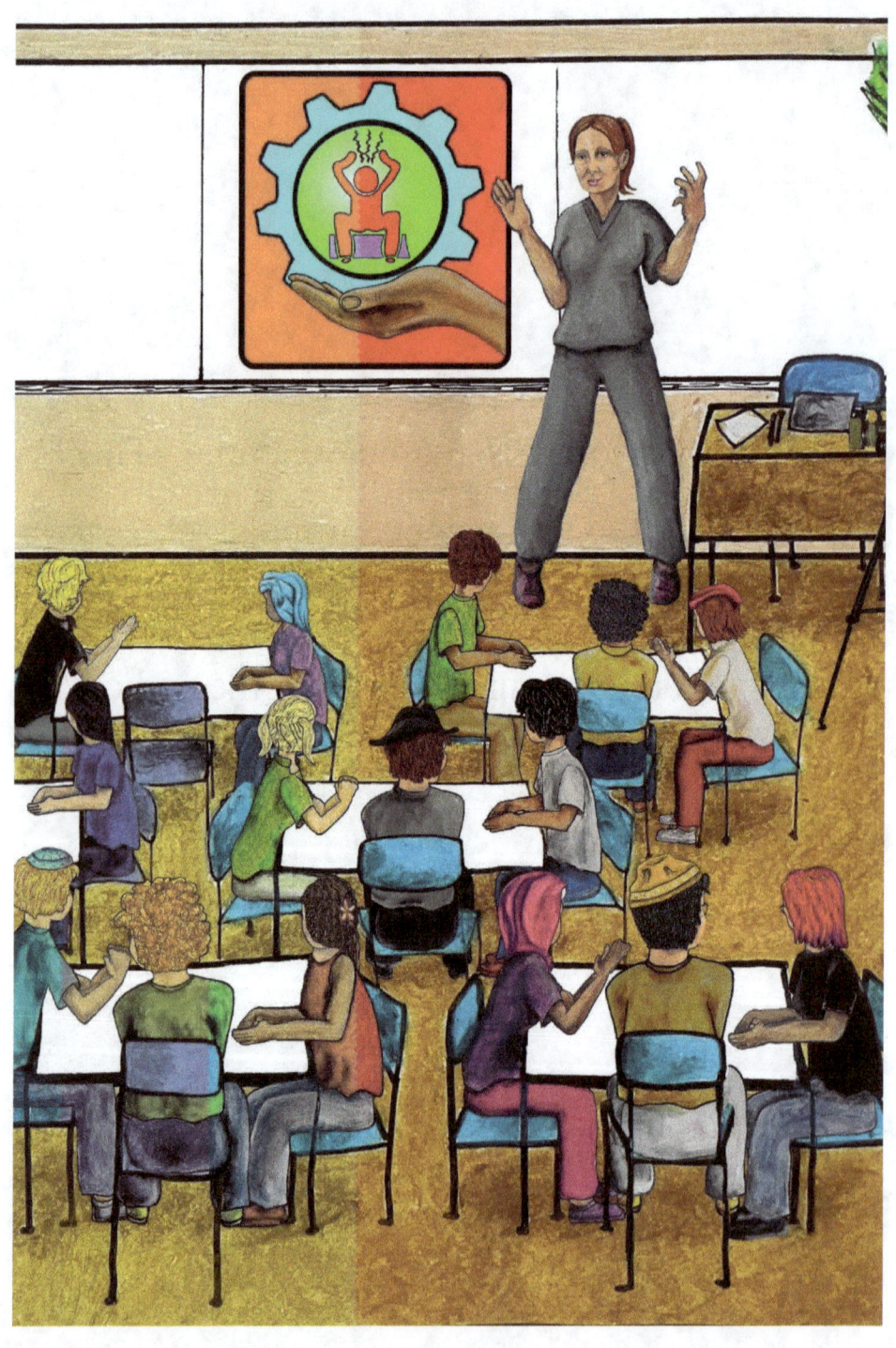

"Anger management is a final example of effortful control. You may get provoked to become angry. Try to pause, think about the consequences of the actions you plan to take, and choose a response that is more helpful to the situation."

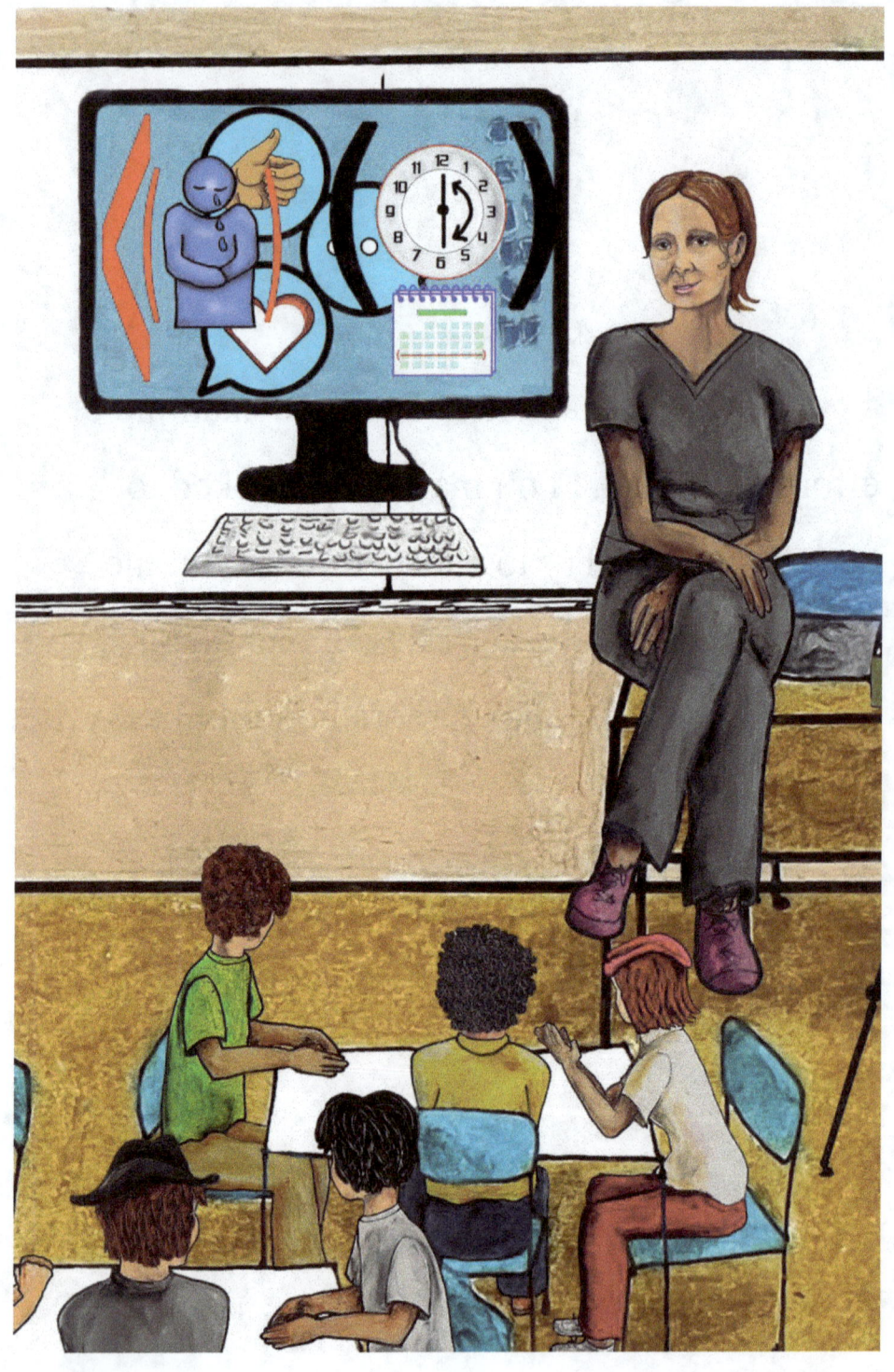

"Now, we're going to talk about tips to help you manage social media. The first is from a research study about limiting social media. The researchers found that if people limited social media use to 30 minutes a week, then they experienced less loneliness and depression."

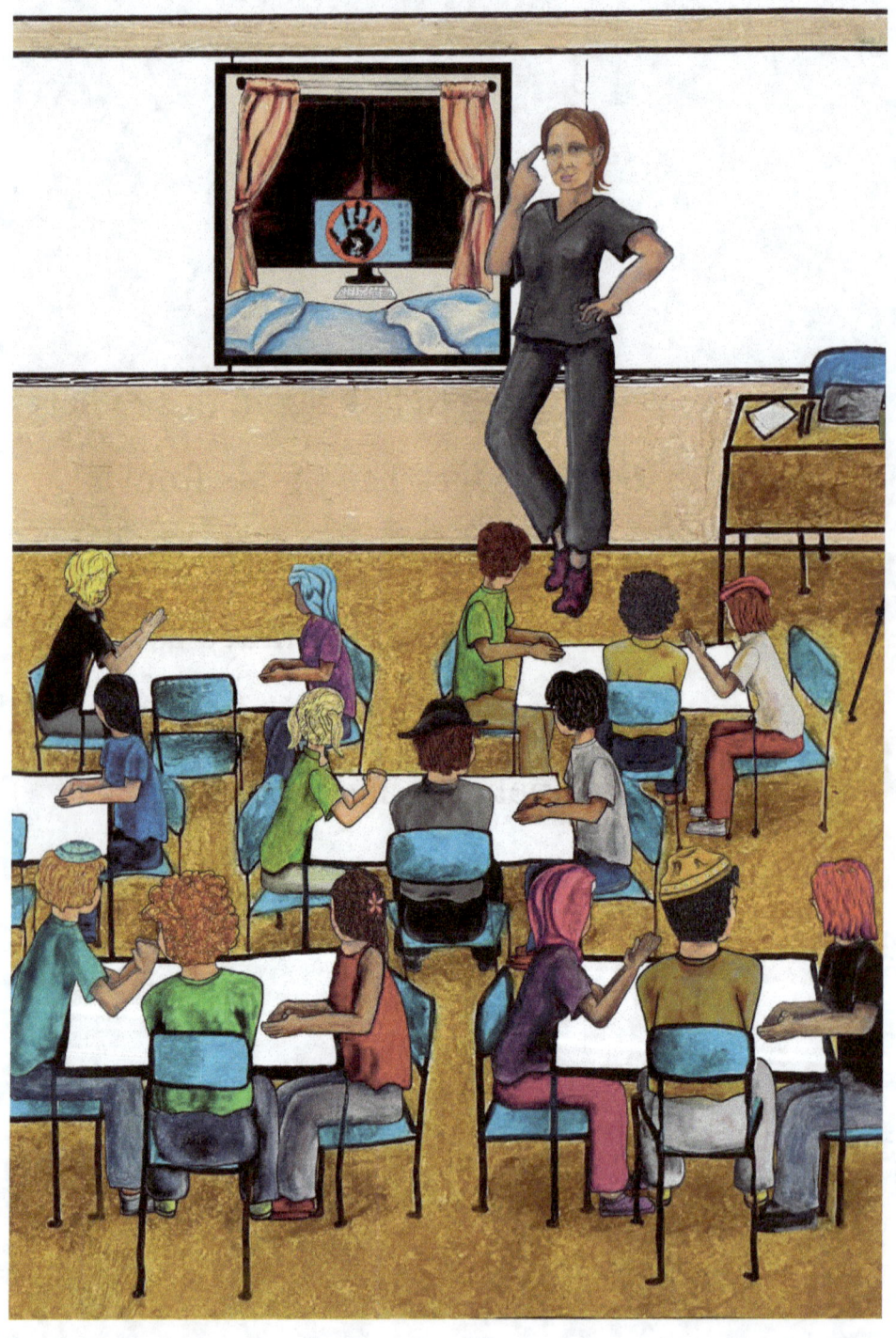

"Research also shows that limiting screen time before bed can help with getting better sleep."

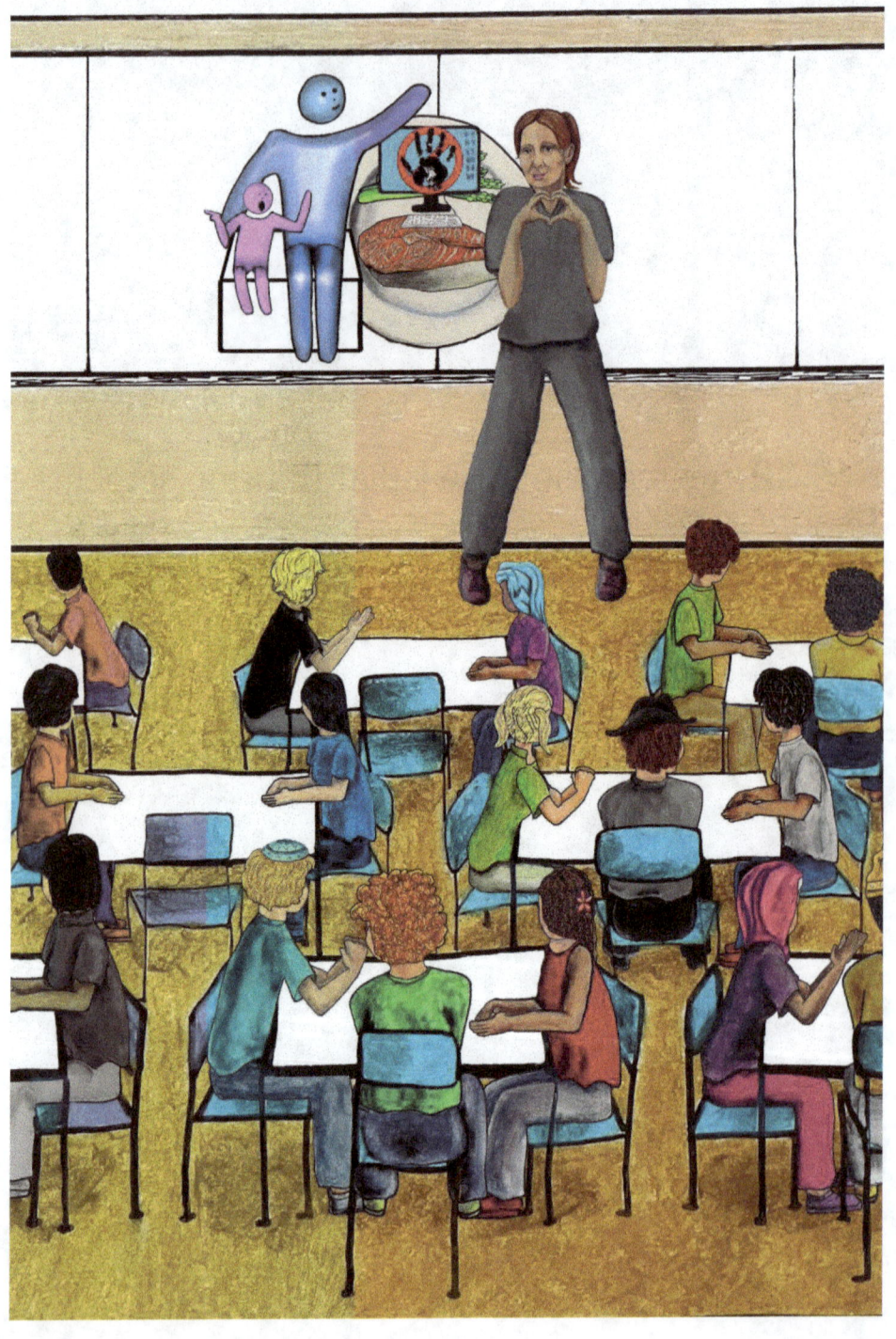

"It is helpful for parents to have regular sit-down times with children to talk about each other's day and other things such as goals for the week, month, or year. It is also helpful if families participate in screen-free meals. Families may want to put their phones and tablets away from the dinner table so that they don't have the opportunity to use their devices."

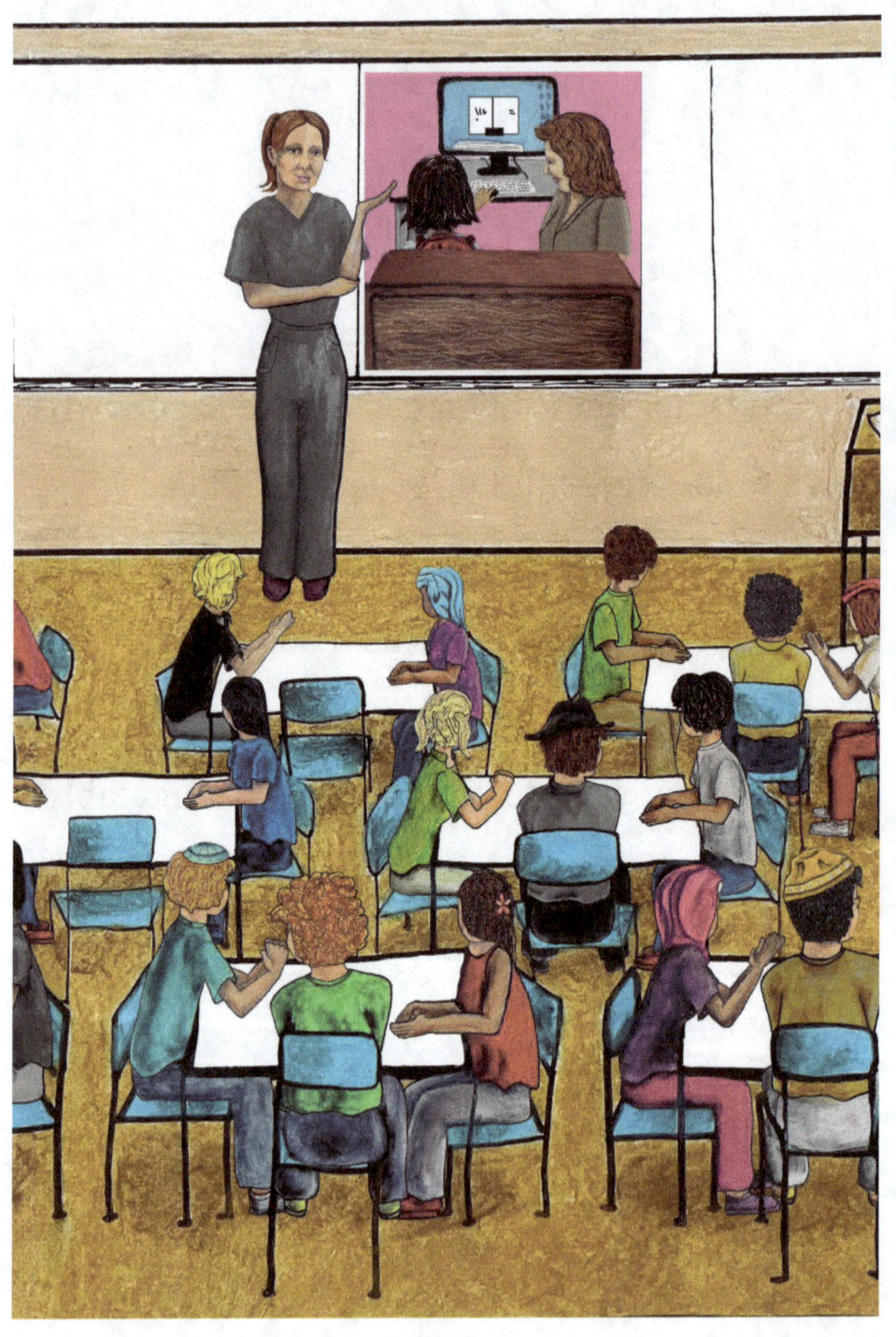

"Another helpful tip for parents is that they should consider learning to play their children's favorite games so that they have another activity to help strengthen family bonds. It's ok for adults to play kid games."

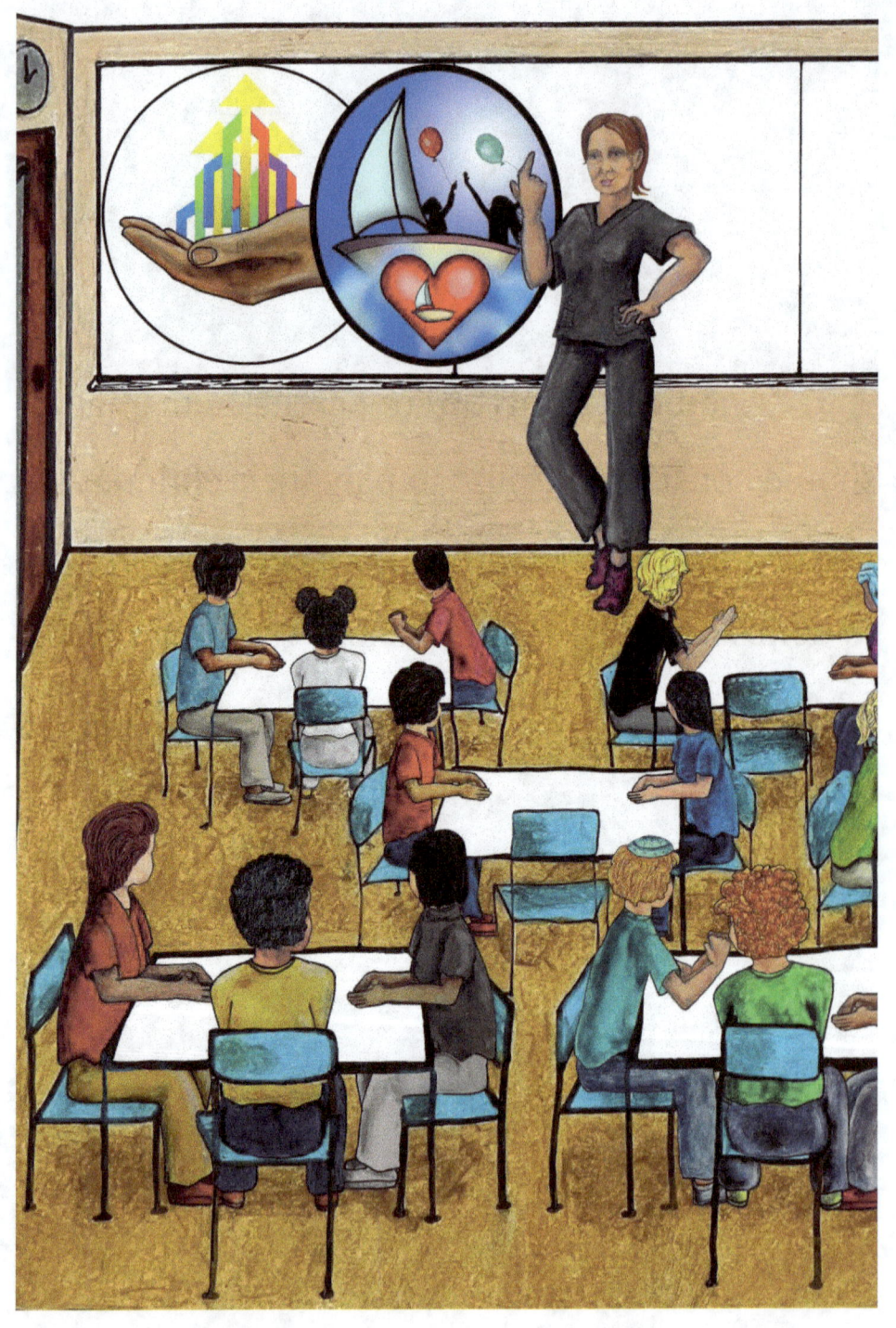

"Parents could also benefit by helping their child plan out time in the week to do the child's favorite things that do not include being online. Having a plan helps to give goals and structure to people's day as well as to set boundaries and limits on how much social media time is spent."

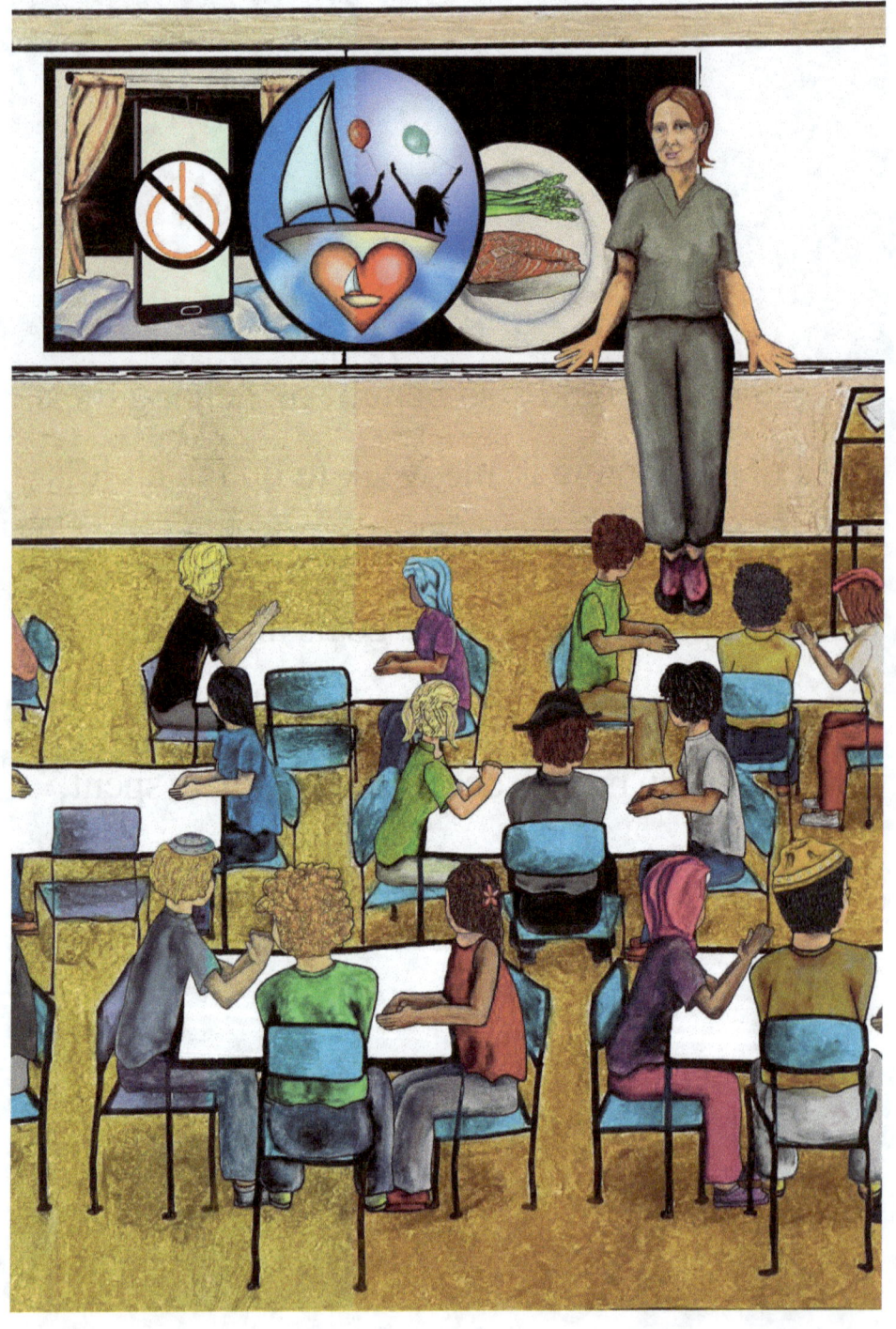

"Another tip is to turn off or silence your phone during family activities. Turning off notifications can help, and people should consider putting their phone on charge outside of their bedroom so they are not tempted to access the device."

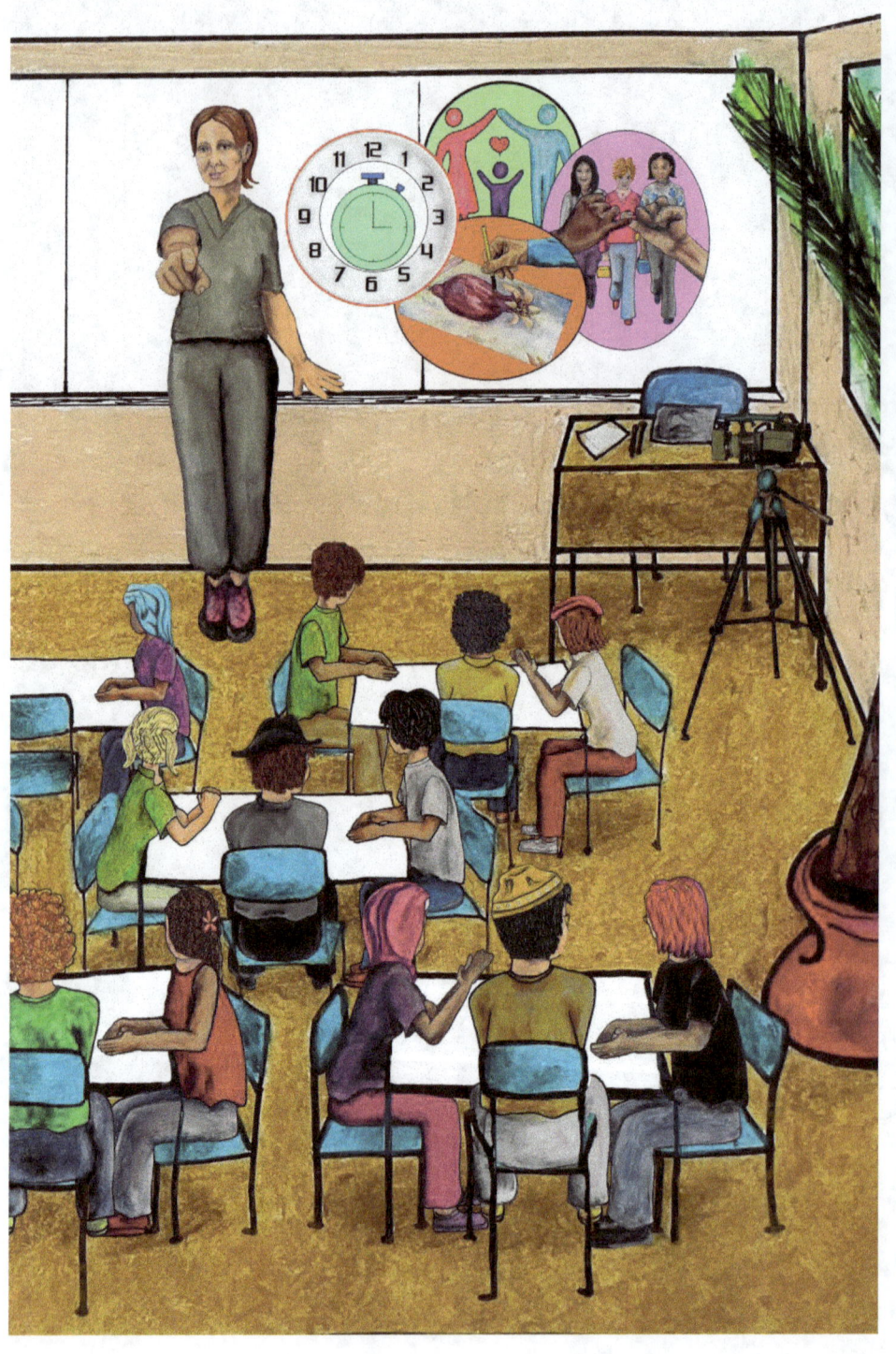

"A person could turn on a timer to help themselves limit their screen usage. People should consider visiting with their family and friends more often in person instead of through social media. If you are finding that you are spending too much time on social media, you may want to consider discovering a new hobby so that you spend your time doing different things."

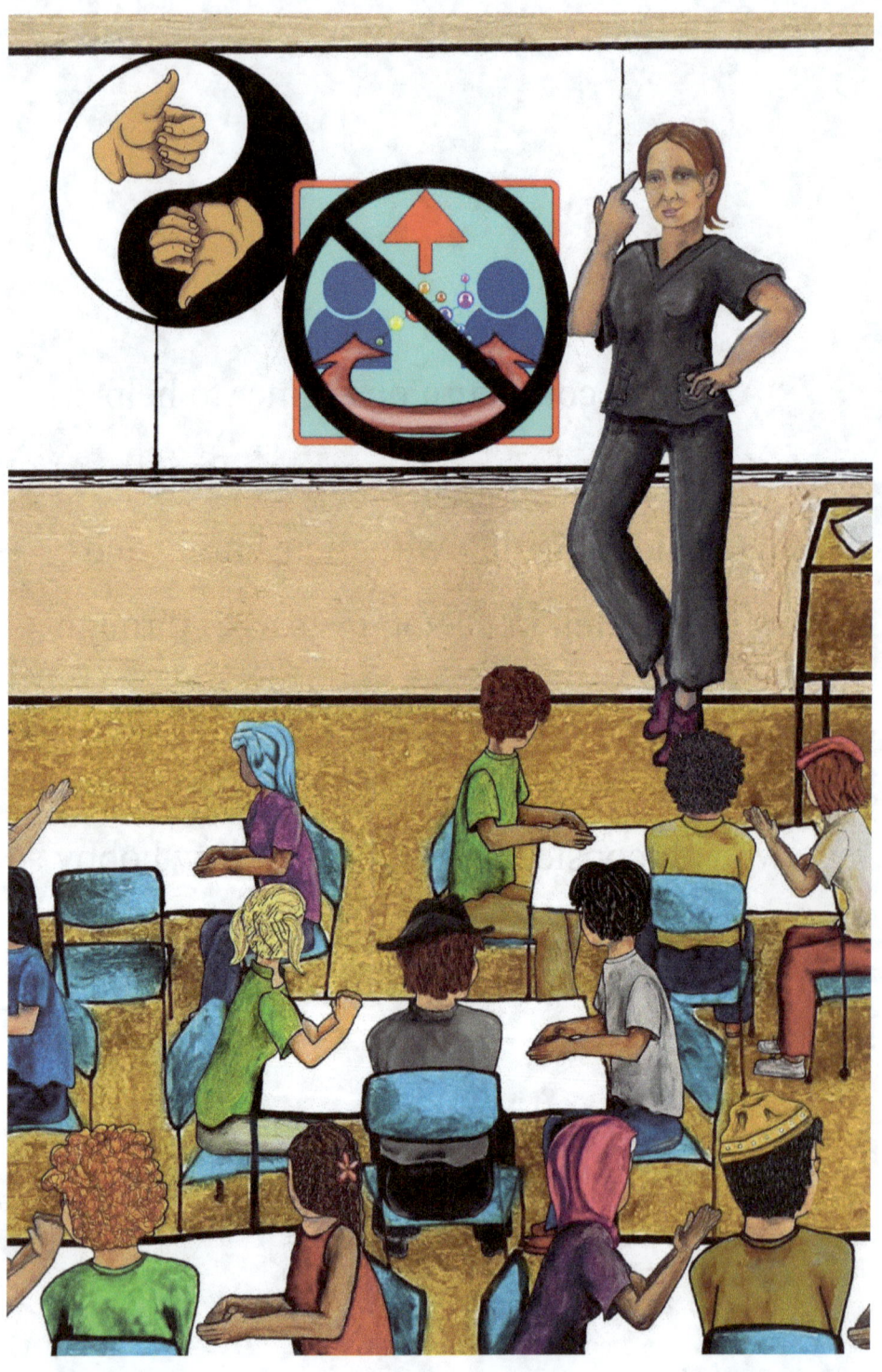

"Remember that most people just post the positive highlights in their life, so try to avoid believing that everyone's life is perfect except yours. That also goes for body images that people may post to try to show beauty and perfection. We are wonderfully made and need to learn the body in which we live. Everyone faces challenges, but not everyone shares them with others. Also, report harassment, hate speech, and threats to moderators or authorities. If you don't know if you should report it, then ask your parents or another trusted adult like a teacher. As others have said, do everything in moderation. Social media is not bad by itself and will be a more useful tool in our lives once we develop better management of our emotions and behaviors."

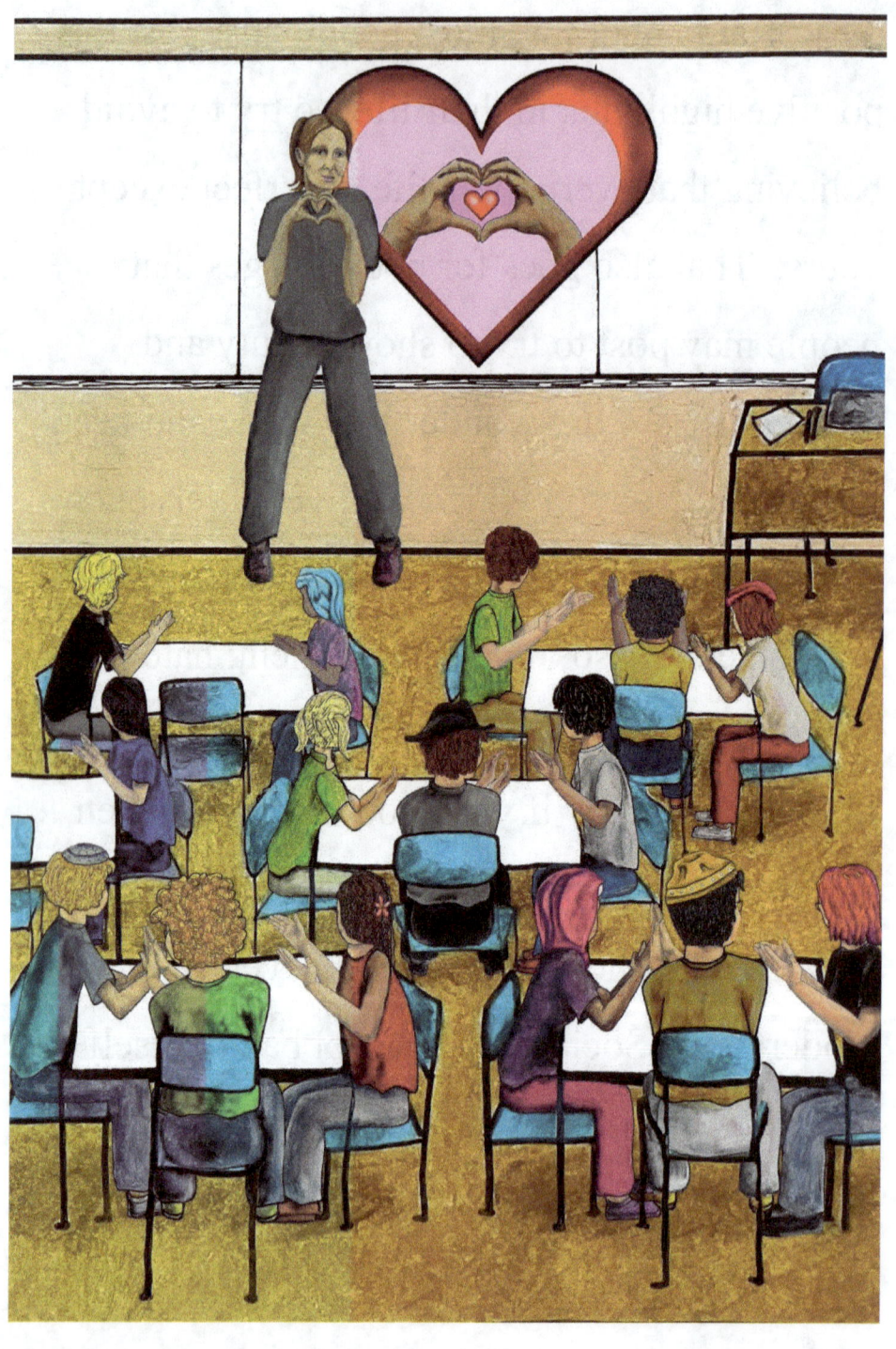

"I want to thank you for attending today's presentation. I hope you learned a lot and will share this information with others. Don't only focus on your own mental health journey, but also help others on their journey to good mental health."

The class starts to clap, and many students say, "Thank you, Nurse Dorothea." Some come up to the nurse after the class is dismissed and give her a big hug telling her how much she helped them.

References

Bekalu, M. A. (2020). Social media use can be positive for mental health and well-being. Retrieved from: https://www.hsph.harvard.edu/news/features/social-media-positive-mental-health/

Brunch, E. (2019). Social Media Isn't Perfect, but It's Brought Us Together in Community, Health, Love, and Beyond. Retrieved from: https://www.wellandgood.com/positive-effects-social-media/

Drew, C. (2023). Effortful Control: Definition, Key Points, Examples. Retrieved from:

https://helpfulprofessor.com/effortful-control/

Drew, C. (2024). 40 Social Media Examples (Ranked by Monthly Users). Retrieved from: https://helpfulprofessor.com/social-media-examples/

Editors of Encyclopedia Britannica. (2024). Social Media. Retrieved from: https://www.britannica.com/topic/social-media

Gudka, M. (2022). How Social Media Can Add to Your Wellbing. Retrieved from: https://theartofhealing.com.au/2022/12/how-social-media-can-add-to-your-wellbeing/

Murphy, E. (2021). Social Media Addiction. Retrieved from: https://recovered.org/addiction/behaviors/social-media-addiction

Naslund, J. A., Bondre, A., Torous, J., & Aschbrenner, K. A. (2021). Social Media and Mental Health: Benefits, Risks, and Opportunities for Research and Practice. *Journal of Technology in Behavioral Science, 2020 Apr 20, 5(3): 245-257.* doi:10.1007/s41347-020-00134-x

Nobel, J. (2018). Does social media make you lonely? Retrieved from: https://www.health.harvard.edu/blog/is-asteady-diet-of-social-media-unhealthy-2018122115600

Patterson, A. (2023). Social Media's Positive Power for Young People. Retrieved from: https://www.psychologytoday.com/us/blog/young-people-decoded/202311/social-medias-positive-power-for-young-people?msockid=1d8695c6a4a56231216d86fda5e963ac

Ruder, D. B. (2019). Screen Time and the Brain. Retrieved from: https://hms.harvard.edu/news/screen-time-brain

Santiago, E. (2024). The 7 Types of Social Media

and Pros & Cons of Each (Research). Retrieved from: https://www.psychologytoday.com/us/blog/young-people-decoded/202311/social-medias-positive-power-for-young-people?msockid=1d8695c6a4a56231216d86fda5e963ac

About the Illustrator

Lindsay acquired her BFA from Columbus College of Art and Design. She was a self-employed metal artist beginning in 1985 and was part of the American Arts and crafts movement of the late 80's and early 90's with an art piece on permanent collection at the White House and the governor's mansion in Ohio. The majority of the works she sold then were done in metal, either soldered or welded. During that time, she spent 5 years serving on the board of Ohio Designer Craftsmen and networked part of her business through them. She sold many of her works through art galleries across the USA and Japan. She did many individual commissions and was also commissioned to do giftware design through Bath and Body Works, i.e., the Limited, in the year 2000.

In 2008, Lindsay went back to college to acquire another degree so she could try her hand at teaching high school art. She acquired a M.Ed. from U of A. She taught art at 6 different schools in AZ before retiring in 2022. In her last 4 years, she taught: Art 1, Advanced Art, AP Art, Ceramics, Advanced Ceramics, and Photography I, II, III, and IV (which was also producing the school's yearbook). Several of her students were recipients of HAA Art scholarships. During her first year of teaching at public schools, she taught Graphic Design. All this time, she enjoyed making art with her students and building her illustration, drawing, and painting skills.

During those teaching years she still accomplished a few commissions of steel sculptures. It started with the first commission from Norton Abrasives of creating the company's mascot. It was a larger-than-life French bulldog named Cooper. Cooper resides at the company's US headquarters in Brownsville TX. The mascot had long lines during one trade show of people wanting to take selfies with it. It was a hit and resulted in a personal commission for a couple in Los Angeles of another bulldog named Sebastian.

When Lindsay retired in 2022, she worked with an old friend in Ohio who is an author and performer on a children's book. All the illustrations in the book including the cover were created by Lindsay. The book is for 0-8 year old children and is called "Sleep Little Raven".

Lindsay has kept a blog since 2008 showing the progress of her works at www.curlycu.com.

In Lindsay's words:
"Making art is like breathing; it is a must for my own survival and sanity."

About the Author

Michael is married to Perla in Tucson, AZ. Michael served in the US Air Force between 2002 and 2010 as an Electronic Warfare Officer on the EC-130H Compass Call and deployed 6 times in the Global War on Terror. Michael then served 8 years as an Army Wounded Warrior Advocate. Michael used his GI bill to go to nursing school and works as an RN at an inpatient psychiatric hospital in Tucson, AZ. Michael enjoys listening to Beethoven and reading a lot of news.

Michael's college education:

B.A. in Psychology from Auburn University,

B.S. in Biology from the University of Alabama at Birmingham,

M.S. in Management from Troy University,

Master in Health Administration from the University of Phoenix,

M.S. from the University of Arizona through the accelerated Master's Entry to the Profession of Nursing program

Other Books by Dow Creative Enterprises®

For more info about Nurse Dorothea books, please visit www.NurseDorothea.com.

Visit www.DowCreativeEnterprises.com for more information about our small publishing company.